NOT
Too Tired to Care

Angela Thomas Jones

Not _Too Tired to Care:_
Learn Evidence-Based Mindfulness Practices to Support Well-being,
Improve Patient Care, and Address the Unique Challenges of These Times

Printed in the United States of America.

ISBN: 978-1-7360221-0-8

Cover Design by 100Covers.com
Interior Design by FormattedBooks.com

Hey, a free gift for YOU!

Panda and I want you to have these *2 FREE GIFTS*
as our way of saying THANKS for buying *NOT* Too Tired to Care

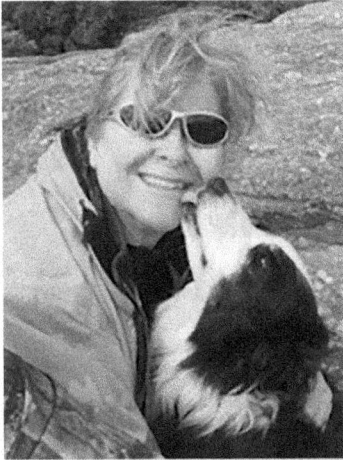

Action Guide Workbook *FREE!*
and
the Turning Point Stories & Transcripts *FREE!*

https://www.nottootiredtocare.com/book

ABOUT THE COVER

Mt. Lafayette, 5249 ft in elevation on the cover, is part
of the Presidential Mountains located in the White
Mountain National Forest of New Hampshire.

Photo by Barry Jones.

Interstate 93 passes through Franconia Notch with Mount Lafayette on the east and Cannon Mountain Ski Area on the west with the Canadian border 70 miles north. Franconia Notch is world-famous for the old man of the mountains also known as the Great Stone Face or the Profile; the geological wonder that inspired Nathaniel Hawthorne to write the Great Stone Face. The Presidential Mountains are part of the Appalachian Mountain range. Thru-hikers on the 2190 mile Appalachian Trail identify the White Mountains of New Hampshire as the most difficult of the entire length from Georgia to Maine. The work culture here is well-suited for tough, independent, *I'll fix it myself and leave me alone, sort of people*—my husband, Barry, and I feel right at home here. We grew up in the southern territory of the Appalachian Mountains and settled in the North Country because of its beautiful rugged-ness and long snowy winters.

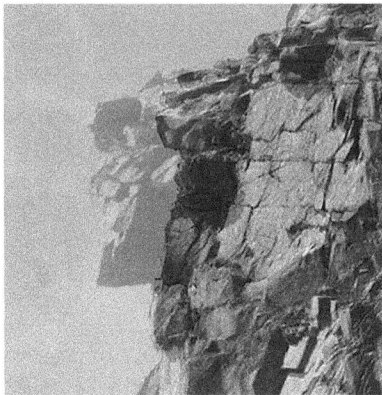

A composite image of the Old Man of the Mountain created from
images taken before and after the collapse on May 3, 2003.

Note the terms 'client', 'patient', 'provider', 'clinician' are used throughout this book. You may use different words depending on your work setting. Please use the language that feels most appropriate for you. Also, Substance Use Disorder (SUD) was adopted by the American Psychological Association in their 2013 revised Diagnostic Statistical Manual as part of a national effort to de-stigmatize the chronic disease of addiction. SUD is used throughout the book as an abbreviation.

CONTENTS

DEDICATION

2020 has been the year for "20/20 hindsight".

This book is dedicated to my trusted colleague and dear friend Karen McNamara, her family, my sisters Kathryn and Cynthia, and all those living with the challenges described in the following true stories.

Karen's words mean more than any expert words on this topic and are the best introduction to the message of the book. She is among the original small group of colleagues who rallied alongside my recovery in 2017 from a close encounter with a plan to end my life by suicide. The conversations that followed evolved into the **North Country Task Force to Improve Opioid Treatment Outcomes by Focusing on Provider Well-being and Resilience.** I know, crazy long title. That same year Karen was the New Hampshire Alcohol and Drug Abuse Counselors Association (NHADACA) Counselor of the Year Nominee. Being nominated for this award is validation of the grace, integrity, and transparency, we, her colleagues, recognized in how she navigated the tragic loss of your son in 2016. Our collective experiences during 2014-2017 were intense, to say the least, and fueled my sense of urgency to find a way out of what at the time felt like an unsolvable dilemma.

Karen's courage to speak honestly about navigating as a clinician and continue with day-to-day stuff that makes up our work-life balance helped me do the same. Our conversations led me to seek answers for how to move forward doing what we love, helping others, and most importantly, without sacrificing our own well-being.

We knew we were onto something when the outcomes of a provider needs assessment she and other colleagues encouraged me to facilitate validated 96% of our colleagues met at risk criteria for compassion fatigue and burnout. What is more, nearly half reported fear of job security loss was keeping them silent with this dilemma. Unacceptable. Since 2016, New Hampshire has been the third hardest hit state in the country with total annual overdose deaths. Unacceptable. This is the reality of our circumstances.

The evidence is indisputable for how chronic stress leads to chronic illness and compromises productivity and quality of care. Self-care is expected as a standard of practice in the work culture of human services. Our code of ethics makes this clear but the work culture of my lifetime has not encouraged speaking openly about these things as demonstrated by the outcomes of our provider needs assessment.

Courageous conversations, advocating for change, and holding ourselves accountable to these standards is what this book is about. This collection of lived experiences is grounded with relevant research and science with the intention of adding to the momentum building across the nation on this topic.

Thanks to the **National Academy of Medicine's Action Collaborative for Clinician Well-Being and Resilience**, they have made it easy to get involved by providing a platform and the resources for building a sustainable and resilient workforce. The rest is up to each of us. This starts with having the conversation about the stuff many are not talking about.

The stories that follow are testimonies of how others are navigating humanity in work-life balance and deliver a message of hope. Karen, thank you for allowing me to share your story along with mine and everyone who has contributed to this journey.

It was March 4, 2016 when my thirty-four-year-old son Jesse Ryan McNamara died from a fentanyl overdose in the town where he grew up and where we still live today. At that time here in the North Country, it had not yet become common knowledge about fentanyl replacing heroin or being mixed with it. The timeline of events is a bit confusing, but I am not surprised due to the intensity of grief packed into a short time. Within a timeframe of about two years 2015–2017 surrounding my son's death, his father and I were facing a horrible divorce, my father died, my precious dog Sasha died, and my mother who lives out of state became terribly ill. I am sure there must have been something else, but this is what comes to mind now.

We managed to get Jesse into treatment twice but there was little local support for recovering heroin addicts at that time in our community. This was at the very beginning of the Recovery Support movement in New Hampshire ("Recovery and Recovery Support"). I was actively working with local resources to form an all recovery group in town with hopes of opening a local Recovery Center in our town where my private practice is also located. My son had some clean time and was doing well. This relapse killed him. He was sold fentanyl expecting heroin. There is still a homicide case pending. There was great confusion over the jurisdiction of his case. He and I had talked about fentanyl and how people were dying because they used it not knowing it was mixed in the heroin they were using.

I remember describing to him with urgency about how lethal it is because of how it shuts down the respiratory system. You know, they just stop breathing. He said "Mom, I'm not stupid! I am careful and only buy from people I know." I think I showed him an obituary of someone I knew and told him, "They weren't stupid either. It happens."

My worst fear came true. *His death was caused by an overdose. I was not prepared for him to die, I mean really, is there any way to be prepared for your child's death? Even if you know the facts, it's just not the way life is supposed to go, so you want to think for the best. I had been working really hard to develop local support for addicts recognizing it was a hidden epidemic at the time. You know how it is as a counselor, we see this stuff day to day in our client's lives and deal with it but when it comes to our children that's a whole different thing.*

Yea, right, we learn about it in ethics class, the boundary stuff, but honestly, you know, living it is when we get it.

The face of heroin addicts has changed *during my lifetime. I've been in long-term recovery over thirty years and working as a Licensed Alcohol and Drug Counselor for over half that time.*

During the past ten years or so I've been seeing cherub-faced college students who were addicted. *Never in my lifetime have I seen this in my years of providing counseling to inmates in jail and prison. I've had many clients at the jail who I believed sincerely wanted to be sober but die shortly after their release due to an overdose. I rarely saw an obituary about these deaths in the newspaper and believe many families must have been shamed from printing the truth.*

I know a family who didn't even have a funeral for their son who died from an overdose.

When Jesse died, his father and I didn't want to hide it. *During that time, where we live, any mention of death by overdose usually included an assumption criminal behavior was involved. My son did not have a criminal record and if he did, why should that matter? I mean really. Jesse was an incredibly special man, loving son, father, brother, and friend to many. We really felt people should have a better understanding for how this can happen to any of us. Our community is so small, it seemed like a simple solution to me…I mean raise awareness by telling the whole truth about our son's death.*

We organized a community event where we live, *the same community where Jesse and his sister grew up and went to school. We hosted a local **Narcan training** and showing of **The Anonymous People**, the 2013 documentary film* *promoting recovery. My daughter and I spoke at this event, sharing our perspective on addiction, recovery, and how Jesse's life and death motivate use to speak up and speak out for recovery. My son's former fiancé who is now in recovery also spoke.*

He had gone to inpatient treatment twice in the past year or so. *I needed to understand how this happened to my son and began looking deeper. After his first time in treatment, he said his counselor told him he could continue drinking alcohol, just not use heroin. He knew that was wrong and had no respect for the treatment there. I've since heard from someone who was there for treatment at that time. They told me Jesse helped him a lot while they were there. I am so grateful to know this. In his second treatment, he was introduced to* **Medication Assisted Therapy** *(MAT) and prescribed* **Vivitrol** *and received it as a monthly shot.*

He said it was like a miracle because for the first time he didn't experience cravings like before. *We could see a difference too, he seemed more confident and less distracted. Unfortunately, it was a new treatment, and its availability was too inconsistent to be effective. For someone experiencing intense cravings, urges, and anxiousness that comes with early sobriety to show up for an appointment expecting the monthly injection and told to wait three or four more days then only to go back to face another delay, well, it's discouraging to say the least. I had heard about this happening from my clients, and, at the time I thought it was their excuse for not making a commitment to treatment, but then, after hearing my son say the same thing, I realized this was actually how treatment was being delivered.*

> **Our decision as a family to go public with the truth about Jesse's death and to educate our community about addiction was probably one of the best things we could have done.**

At the time it just seemed like a no-brainer, you know, to tell the truth. *The momentum from that event led to creating a Recovery Support Center in our town. We held weekly Narcotics Anonymous (N.A.) meetings and all recovery meetings. People seemed to come out of the woodwork for these meetings. It was encouraging. But it became hard for me to listen to young men in the N.A. meetings. To see the pain and hear their desperation I would end up feeling like I can never help them enough. Then I started thinking I failed my son. This is not productive for me. So, I started reducing my amount of exposure to that and joined the Board of Directors of another Recovery Center out of town to distance myself from these triggers. I still have a passion to provide help for addicts and still seeking out how to do that without direct involvement like I have been in my career as a therapist and counselor.*

There is so much more work to be done to educate people about the disease of addiction not just the general public but also in the healthcare system itself.

Find the rest of Karen's story in the Turning Point Stories and Transcripts.

FOREWORD

by Dr. Arthur Hengerer, MD

I grew up in a medical family environment and followed that path to have a 45-year career in various aspects of medical education, administration, clinical practice, and lastly regulation. It has afforded me the opportunity to see and experience the wonderful rewards of medicine, as well as the impact it had both personally and for others from the stress, system pressures, and choices required. At times, the results were the development of mental health issues or addictions and clinicians avoided treatment because of the stigma associated with the perception of showing weakness or fear of jeopardizing their license to practice. In this Forward, the term "clinician" will refer to all those in the health professions impacted by burnout, addiction, and now the pandemic.

My personal interest in this issue derives from years of offering support and guidance to many physicians in obvious distress, burned out, sustaining moral injury or addiction. I also faced times where my own workload in patient care and non-aligned system requirements led to poor decisions about my health and well-being that negatively impacted my work/life balance. This influenced two critical decisions and periods in my life. First, is revisiting my first marriage and the failed responsibilities managing my work/life balance, the lack of personal involvement and behaviors in the relationship, and selfish decisions that ultimately ended in a divorce. Second, was when I needed to spend an extended period of time caring for a spouse who ultimately lost her life after a long battle with cancer.

As I reflect on those two relationships, I realize how fragile I had become and what this meant in terms of potential risks to my health and welfare, family commitments, and the many patients under my care. Ultimately, I was lucky enough to recognize those times of need to address my well-being and sought help to both assess and improve my total fitness. I count myself fortunate in this regard, particularly as I look back on a career in medicine where some of my colleagues and friends did not come to the same recognition and consequently were not as lucky. This book, "NOT Too Tired to Care," helped me to better understand the commitment and rewards I have received from being involved in supporting many burned out and troubled clinicians.

Over the past 10 years this inspired me to transition from clinical practice to become involved with how medicine and health care is governed and organized. I was fortunate enough to have been appointed to serve on our state medical board, which enabled me to better understand the role of medical licensure and discipline in patient safety and public protection. It also created opportunities to become involved with the Federation of State Medical Boards (FSMB), The National Academy of Medicine (NAM), and Federation of State Physician Health Programs (FSPHP) in a variety of responsibilities.

It is the notion that a major barrier to clinicians seeking care for their personal health and, specifically mental health issues, including burnout and depression, was the probing and intrusive nature of the questions asked by state licensing boards on initial licensure applications and renewals. The origin and rationale for such questions on licensing applications comes from a perspective of patient protection so the intensity of questions fluctuated with timing and by the different state boards. The aim is to identify possible risk to patient safety resulting from impairment affecting the clinicians' ability to provide safe care. The clinicians' concern is the impact of a positive response to certain questions including seeking care for one's mental health or a given diagnosis and/or distant past history can create. Positive responses could potentially lead to excessive investigation, burdensome restrictions on the clinician's ability to practice, or even outright denial of a license and disruption or termination of a career. This may make clinicians reluctant to answer these questions honestly. In fact, it has become evident the providers will not only submit false or fraudulent applications, but will also avoid seeking the help they need or elect to be treated in a private undisclosed setting, treat themselves, or not receive treatment at all. Thus, while these questions were crafted with the intent to create safety and transparency for the licensing board and public of the clinician's health status, it has resulted in additional and more significant risks to the public; and the clinicians themselves. Worse still, these risk factors are being knowingly hidden and allowed to grow in seriousness until they materialize at a level harmful to patients or clinicians.

Reviewing the Americans with Disabilities Act (ADA) as it relates to mental health questioning, as well as the recent recommendations of the American Psychiatric Association (APA) and the FSMB, they provide specific guidance for phrasing licensing questions. They focus solely on impairment, under care, that is meaningful in the context of the ability to provide safe treatment to patients, rather than looking simply at a condition or past diagnosis.

The licensing community is not alone in its efforts. I have participated in The National Academy of Medicine's (NAM) action collaborative, which has brought together 55 organizations from all segments of the healthcare environment to focus on provider wellness and resilience. In addition, more than 140 health systems have added their support to the effort. We need the involvement of the health care systems and regulators to consider the role they play in the intensity of burnout, addiction, and mental health. It has been shown that taking steps to find resilience and adjusting work/life balance to deal with a dysfunctional work environment does not lead to a happy and healthy workforce or correct the issues we have been discussing.

Clinicians must look to their core values and find ways to adhere to the challenges they face in the health system or they cannot maintain their personal health. That is why the effort that is occurring in the North Country Task Force in New Hampshire under the direction of Angela Thomas Jones and her colleagues is so important. It demonstrates what needs to be accomplished not only nationally but at the local levels to assist in managing addiction issues that will likely be compounded by the Covid-19 pandemic effects. Mother Teresa once said, "I alone cannot change the world. But I can cast a stone across the waters to create many ripples." This book will not be a quick fix to these problems in today's complex health care delivery system but offers a guide and inspiration to all those working on the challenges we face.

Dr. Arthur Hengerer, MD
Co-lead on the National Academy of Medicine Action Collaborative for the Conceptual Model for the Culture of Silence
Former Co-lead on the National Academy of Medicine Action Collaborative for the Conceptual Model Group
Former Chairperson for Board of the Federation of State Medical Boards (FSMB)

FOREWORD

by Roger Carroll

I'd like to think I would know if there is a downside to going public about fighting a mental illness.

Admittedly, I don't always know what I don't know, but in November 2018 I sat outside a gun shop and seriously contemplated taking my life. My emotional pain had become that unbearable.

Instead, I drove to a therapy appointment where, based on my behavior and demographic, I entered the New Hampshire mental health system.

I was parked in an emergency room for more than 24 hours while I waited for a bed to become available at one of the designated receiving facilities in the state that treat people with mental illness. I spent five days at the Designated Receiving Facility (DRF) under the care of an amazing group of doctors and nurses.

I still had a lot of work to do after I was released, but I also had a strong support system. My wife, daughter, and family stood by me as I knew they would, but less certain was how the people at work would react.

When I called my boss from the DRF and told him where I was, he was nothing but supportive. My first day back on the job I told my staff. It was clear that not only did none of them think less of me for seeking the help I needed, they respected me for it.

As word of my hospitalization got out in our small office, others came up to me and shared words of support, sometimes accompanied by hints that my struggle hit home with them.

Then I did something that might be considered foolish or crazy according to the conventional wisdom surrounding mental health as something to be talked about only in whispers: I decided to write about the experience.

One person who worked in health care reacted to the idea like I had just told her of my intention to go over Niagara Falls in a laundry basket. I chalked that up to the ethic of the medical profession that held mental health as something not to be openly talked about.

The three part series, "A journey through New Hampshire's mental health system," was published at the end of December. It appeared in newspapers across the state, and was posted on multiple Twitter feeds and Facebook timelines.

The emails, texts, Facebook comments, Twitter messages, and phone calls I received numbered in the hundreds. People stopped me on the street to shake my hand and tell me how much they appreciated what I wrote. Many poured out their hearts in emails and shared stories about their battles with mental illness, or those of a family member. Some voiced their frustrations with the system, and they all—to a person—thanked me for coming forward. There wasn't a single negative comment in the bunch, and I have not detected that people treat me differently since I told my story.

I never felt stigmatized by seeking help or going public about my journey, though I've occasionally wondered why people reacted in the ways they did. The answer, I think, is a fairly simple but universal truth: People respond to honesty.

Roger Carroll,
Manager Editor
Laconia Daily Sun and Co-founder Granite State News Collaborative, New Hampshire

INTRODUCTION

This book is about work-life balance motivated from my Therapy Dog Panda and my lived experience. The purpose of this book is to contribute to efforts already under way to break the silence in our health care work culture that expects more for less therefore promoting self-sacrifice. I hope it will inspire you to do the same.

Changing a cultural norm requires steady and diligent advocacy. This book is an outcome of courageous and compassionate conversations among colleagues, friends, and family. These courageous conversations became a small grassroots movement now part of a National Call to Action for Clinician Well-Being and presented in three sections. The full transcripts of the interviews are available in the **Turning Point Stories & Transcripts**. Each chapter includes an invitation for reflection and action related to the concepts presented. **An Action Guide Workbook** includes each of the reflection activities found in each chapter with a robust resource list.

Part One: The Precious 20% establishes the foundation for this topic based on evidence from validated study. Lived experience told through Turning Point stories and interviews illustrate the key for maintaining resilience is feeling effective at what we do. **For health and human service professionals, this is called compassion satisfaction**. According to evidence-based research, we need a minimum 20% of our total workload to meet criteria for compassion satisfaction to keep burnout at bay.

The question is, *how* we achieve and maintain this
precious 20% while working in chaos and uncertainties
that come with epidemics and global pandemic.

Addressing this question is the focus of this book.

The first Turning Point story is from the Medical Director of the New Hampshire Professionals Health Program (NHPHP). Her story describes experiences influencing her choice to dedicate her career to this non-profit organization with the sole purpose of encouraging the well-being and recovery of New HampshireHealthcare Professionals through compassion, education, advocacy, and hope.

Part Two. Introducing Solutions: The Biology of Stress and the Science of Hope. Turning Point stories and interviews share how thriving beyond the precious 20% is possible and sustainable. You will learn a simple four-step trauma-sensitive and evidence-informed practice called HomeBase. This self-care practice is a tool you can use anywhere, anytime, and is appropriate to teach your clients, peers, friends, and family. I developed HomeBase while working for the Department of Corrections and share the story of how it got its name and why it is effective at building sustainable resilience, the science of hope.

Part Three: Where Rubber Meets Pavement is about advocacy. This section opens with an introduction from Linda Massimilla, New Hampshire State Representative of the North Country. During my term on the Board of Directors of the New Hampshire Alcohol and Drug Abuse Counselors Association (NHADACA), we updated the scope of the Ethics Committee to reflect a more clear commitment to Clinician Well-Being and became the first professional organization in New Hampshireto join the National Academy of Medicine Call to Action for Clinician Well-Being. Instructions for how to become a Network Organization and why this is important are included.

I hope this material brings you insight, understanding,
maybe a laugh or two, and something useful.

"The first step of a thousand miles starts with a single step."
Lao Tzu

PART ONE

The Precious 20%

> "The only thing we have is one another. The only competitive advantage we have is the culture and values of the company. Anyone can open up a coffee store. We have no technology, we have no patent. All we have is the relationship around the values of the company and what we bring to the customer every day. And we all have to own it."
>
> **Howard Schultz, CEO, Starbucks**

Introduction to the problem. Burnout.

> "Be kinder to yourself. And then let your kindness flood the world."
>
> *Pema Chodron*

Quote contributed by Rebecca Libby, MS
School Counselor for the Manchester School District
Adjunct Professor, Southern New Hampshire University, Psychology Department
Go to the Turning Point Stories & Transcripts to find Rebecca's full story and interview.

CHAPTER ONE PREVIEW

This chapter establishes the foundation for exploring the burnout dilemma healthcare workers and SUD treatment providers are facing right now. In this chapter, burnout is defined and described through lived experience that motivated a small grassroots movement in the North Country of New Hampshire and joined the National Academy of Medicine's Action Collaborative on Clinician Well-Being and Resilience ("Action Collaborative"). For the purposes of the discussion explored in this book, the dilemma is identified as to how to continue providing quality care during uncertain times and remain healthy enough to not only *survive* these challenges but continue finding joy and meaning in our work. It is important to also recognize the burnout dilemma has multiple contributing factors. I believe two primary factors are ourselves as individuals and the industry of the healthcare work culture. The responsibilities of each are addressed, however, with focus on the responsibility we bring, as individuals, to this equation. **"The precious 20%"** is a term I use to migrate meaning from research indicating an 80/20 ratio as the baseline for preventing professional burnout (Shanafelt, "Executive

Leadership" and "Career Fit"). These two numbers represent one hundred percent of the workload for healthcare professionals. The larger number represents the required daily administrative and operational tasks. The smaller number is the percentage where meaning and purpose are experienced. This part involves the relationships with our clients and patients, their families, and our work colleagues. Because of the nature of this relational value, it holds the most power in the equation and is the reason I call it "the precious 20%". The Professional Quality of Life measure defines the meaningful and fulfilling part of our work as compassion satisfaction and suggests this is the key factor for determining our ability to *thrive* and remain resilient (Stamm). Surviving is a short-term response for white knuckling it through a crisis. I purposefully use the word *thriving* rather than *surviving* because I believe compassion satisfaction is the essence of thriving. Work-life balance is used throughout the book when referring to that which is our own responsibility in this dilemma. The question is ***how to harness this precious 20% of compassion satisfaction so we can maintain resilience for the long haul.***

In 2016, New Hampshire was hit hard by what the U.S. Surgeon General identified as Addiction: A National Epidemic *("Facing Addiction")*.

Since then, New Hampshirehas remained third to West Virginia and Ohio with the highest number of deaths due to Opioid overdoses despite being one of the states with the smallest population. During that same year, on separate occasions, two trusted colleagues shared with me, in confidence, their thoughts about not renewing their license to practice as SUD treatment providers.

We had worked together in various capacities for three decades. I know these two individuals to be "solid" professionals and have never seen them back down from a challenge. The constant rise in the rates of relapse and overdose deaths in their caseloads had become overwhelming. Barriers among other care providers due to misinformation, negative judgements about people with substance use disorders, or lack of coordination seemed to have become the norm. Both said they no longer felt effective and could not see any other solution. They described feeling no longer connected with the joy of their work and a sense of not caring anymore because of the non-stop sense of crisis and little evidence of change.

Compromises in patient care and safety were being made daily on a regular basis. I saw this firsthand. At the time, I believed I could make a difference as the Clinical Director of one of New Hampshire's Substance Use Disorder

Treatment Centers. The overwhelming need for substance use disorder treatment in our community plus the frustration of constantly turning people away because of long waitlists felt relentless. For myself, the reality of these barriers began to sink in when I learned about the closing of one of the primary referral sources in our region. This facility had a long-established reputation of being a caring and effective provider of inpatient and outpatient Substance Use Disorder treatment. What is more, the closing was due to inability of the staff to maintain safe care.

The newspapers reported several complaints were filed with the State Department of Health and Human Services. The complaints were said to be written by employees working at the facility as well as clients and their family members. After weeks of investigation, the Board of Directors of that facility published their announcement to close the facility because they could not see a resolution due to the workforce shortage of qualified professionals. This was a concrete affirmation of demand exceeding resources and marked the beginning of my own journey on a similar path my two trusted colleagues had described.

---

*7 For the first time, the World Health Organization (WHO) classifies workplace **burnout as an occupational phenomenon**.

The WHO says it is a syndrome

resulting from chronic workplace stress that has not been successfully managed.

The WHO previously defined burnout as a "state of vital exhaustion," but this is the first time it's being directly linked in its classification of diseases **as a work hazard** (ICD-10).

---

*7 According to Dan Schawbel, research director at Human Resource advisory firm Future Workplace, the syndrome of burnout is now an "epidemic" and he expects the issue to worsen. He says burnout is causing more employees than ever to contact their health services provider or their Human Resource Department at work for a reason other than an illness or health condition.

Burnout is characterized by:

> feelings of energy depletion or exhaustion
> increased mental distancing from one's job,
or feelings of negativism or
> cynicism related to one's job; and reduced professional efficacy.

The term "burnout"
was coined in the 1970s by American psychologist
Herbert Freudenberger. He used it to describe
the consequences of severe stress and
high ideals in "helping" professions ("Depression").

A few months later, one of these colleagues told me she could not see these circumstances improving. I will never forget the look of loss in her eyes at that moment when she said, "I can't do this anymore." After talking through several scenarios, she confided she had bought a gun with the intention of ending her life by suicide. I knew her to be knowledgeable of handling a firearm, as are many in the North Country, and knew she was serious.

After sitting in silence together for what felt like an eternity, I will never forget my feeling of utter helplessness when she asked, "Should I talk with the Licensing Board about this?" Our Licensing Board was the furthest thing on my mind at that moment. All I could say was something like, "What could they do?" My colleague gave me a smirk and commented, "Well, who the hell do I go to with this!?" Together we worked out a plan for getting through the next twenty-four hours. I promised I would research her question about speaking with the Licensing Board.

> That moment was the beginning of my quest to understand not only how to effectively respond to the question of provider impairment but also how to sensitively manage the risks impairment introduces to client care.

At that time, it never occurred to me the following year I would mirror their footsteps. I am happy to say both of us continue to work through the challenges of our work and are thriving in our work-life balance.

Her courage continues to inspire my own journey in the process of navigating work-life balance during these uncertain times. When I asked her how she felt about fully disclosing her name and her story she didn't hesitate to say, "Yes, of course...all of us need to talk more about this stuff...how else is anything going to change?"

Find Karen McNamara's full Turning Point Story
and update in the Transcripts.

During the past several years researching this topic, I found most validated studies regarding healthcare provider burnout involve emergency response personnel, physicians, nurses, and medical practice interns. The following information was taken from resources provided by the National Academy of Medicine (NAM) Action Collaborative on Clinician Well-Being and Resilience.

Clinicians of all kinds, across all specialties and care settings, are experiencing alarming rates of burnout. Among the most telling of statistics, more than 50 percent of U.S. physicians report significant symptoms. Burnout is a syndrome characterized by a high degree of emotional exhaustion and depersonalization (i.e., cynicism), and a low sense of personal accomplishment at work.

*Clinician burnout can have serious, wide-ranging consequences, from reduced job performance and high turnover rates to—in the most extreme cases—**medical error and clinician suicide.** On the other hand, clinician well-being supports improved patient-clinician relationships, a high-functioning care team, and an engaged and effective workforce. In other words, when we invest in clinician well-being, everyone wins.*

> *400 physicians die by suicide per year, which is two times greater than that of the general population* (Mealer).
>
> **7 More than one physician dies by suicide per day in the US.*

Supporting clinician well-being requires sustained attention and action at organizational, state, and national levels, as well as investment in research and information-sharing to advance evidence-based solutions.

Burnout does not just negatively affect workers. A 2017 study says 95% of human resource leaders say the syndrome sabotages workplace retention. The WHO also noted that burnout prevents professional success ("The Employee Burnout Crisis").

The research I found regarding burnout for behavioral health providers is dated, but worth sharing; perceived clarity of the role of the team, personal role clarity, identification with one's profession and the team, case-load size and composition were identified as contributing factors for emotional exhaustion, low personal accomplishment, depersonalization, job satisfaction, and sick leave among community mental health teams that were examined.

Because of the above-mentioned factors, mental health specialists are at high risk for burnout. Burnout levels of up to 40% have been reported in the U.S. psychologists (Onyett). The following table is taken from *Overcoming Compassion Fatigue: A Practical Resilience Workbook* by Teater & Ludgate (2017).

Compassion fatigue in different professional groups

Professional Group	Approximate Incidence of Problem
Health care workers	16-85%
Emergency room nurses	33% met criteria 85% symptoms in past week
Hospice workers	34%
Paramedics	25% and above

Incidence of burnout in different groups

Population	Approximate incidence of problem
Working adults in general	13-27.8%
Mental health/occupational therapists	54%
Psychologists	Up to 40%
Childcare workers	50%
Clergy	40% mild to severe
Medical doctors in general	37.9-45.8%

In the Introduction of this Workbook, co-author Martha Teater uses the metaphor of air travel emergency procedure instructions for "putting the provided oxygen mask on first then helping others." This is a great metaphor for self-care and provider well-being. We must first take care of ourselves so we may help others. John Ludgate describes the loss of respected colleagues to suicide. He describes these colleagues as international experts on the topic of self-care and acknowledges the questions I found myself asking: How can this happen without recognizing it before it is too late? How can we sensitively respond?

Reading this introduction to their workbook validated my quest for answers. John Ludgate's honesty about the loss of his two colleagues to death by suicide and how this influenced his decision to co-author the workbook inspired me. More importantly, I felt less alone and encouraged.

According to data available
on the American Association of Suicidology website,
suicide is:

10th leading cause of death in the U.S.
2nd leading cause of death for ages 15 - 34

1 person dies by suicide every 10.9 minutes
1 male every 13.9 minutes and 1 female every 49.7 minutes
1 attempt every 26 seconds
25 attempts for every death by suicide
1 of every 61 Americans is a survivor of suicide loss

As many as 40-50% of the population
have been exposed to suicide in their lifetime (Drapeau).

Each day, an average of 20 veterans die by suicide
("Protecting Veterans' Access").

From Tonya Taveres interview: *From my perspective, there should be no stigma (or guilt) attached to compassion fatigue—it is incredibly challenging to continually face trauma alongside others and try to help people out of their darkest times. We have much work to do on this front. Nor should there be stigma or guilt attached to wanting to excel in our work but maintain a balanced life.*

I think having open and honest discussions about the reality of compassion fatigue, what that means, root causes, what it looks like, and how it manifests for people is incredibly important. Equally important is to understand what compassion satisfaction is, looks like, and feels like for the team. What things are important to each person, and what helps them to feel better. Knowing these things helps me to better prepare to have appropriate tools in place, have critical conversations at the right times, promote well-being and lead by example, and offer opportunities to learn and practice resiliency building skills.

Some practical ways to promote this that I feel work well include giving staff and team members opportunities to take ownership in their work and roles, providing them chances to feel more connected to their work, revived, and successful. It's important to also highlight and celebrate successes, no matter how big or small, and do it in ways that honor yourself and your staff, i.e., find out how people like to be praised and what type of feedback works for them (some people like grand gestures and spotlights on them, while for others this can be very uncomfortable).

Global Pandemic has pushed the topic of burnout and provider well-being to the top of the list of national discussion. This will continue to motivate collection of data relevant not only for the treatment and preventive care associated with COVID-19, but the ripple effects as well.

During July 2020, I had the pleasure of speaking with Rebecca Etz, PhD, of the Larry A. Green Center in Virginia about the data they are collecting. She explained how she and her colleagues at the Larry A. Green center hatched the idea of a nation-wide survey to track adaptations and associated impact on primary care systems. You can access their weekly posts by visiting their website described below.

On March 13, 2020,

the Larry A. Green Center in Virginia
partnered with the Primary Care Collaborative

and launched a weekly national survey to better understand the response and capacity of US primary care practices to COVID-19, as well as the potential impact of the pandemic on primary care.

The "Quick COVID-19 Primary Care Survey" occurs weekly. Each survey takes less than 3 minutes to complete and includes 4 core questions and a "flash" question. Suggestions for flash questions are always accepted—they are designed to respond to the most pressing information needs.

A new survey and link are generated each Friday at 9am EST and closes each Monday at 11:59pm PST. Survey invitations are distributed with the help of professional societies and organizations, listservs, and practice-based research networks. Invitations include links to the most recent survey findings. Each survey offers participants the option to sign up for an automated mailing to receive the new link each week directly, thanks to the assistance of our partner TechNeed.

In response to the announcement of Global Pandemic, The National Academy of Medicine posted this statement on their website: *In the face of the unprecedented challenges created by the COVID-19 pandemic and the accompanying global public health emergency, the Action Collaborative on Clinician Well-Being and Resilience must acknowledge the toll that the current crisis is taking on the well-being of clinicians. We know that the health care and public health community needs our support as they navigate the difficult challenges arising in this unprecedented moment. We have therefore compiled a list of strategies and resources to support the health and well-being of clinicians providing health care during the COVID-19 outbreak (National Academy of Medicine).* Find NAM's contact information in the Resource section at the back of the book.

Invitation for Reflection and Action

If you are one of those 61 people who knows someone who died by suicide, take a moment to pause.

If you are not one of those 61 people and do not personally know anyone who has died by suicide, take a moment to pause.

If you wish, consider the insight you have gained from this experience.

In response, what act of kindness can you give yourself in this moment?

Several months after the courageous conversations, I attended an Ethics training. This training was designed for mental health and substance use disorder treatment professionals. I do not recall the exact title of the training, but I do remember it mentioned risk management for clinicians to avoid complaints being filed against their practice and that was what I wanted to hear about.

The first part of the presentation included discussion about existing risk management mechanisms. It was during this discussion I began thinking about what is predictable is preventable, or, as my maternal grandmother would say, "An ounce of prevention is worth a pound of cure."

In this case, **prevention** is the health and well-being
of health care workers and **the problem is compromised**
patient care and safety due to provider fatigue and burnout.

The Ethics presentation was delivered by a New Hampshire Attorney. Their practice specializes in representing behavioral health clinicians under investigation by the licensing board that govern their license to practice. I had heard about her practice through word of mouth and wanted to learn for myself what this attorney might have to offer. This training was an opportunity to do that and collect continuing education credits required for my license retention—a win-win.

More importantly, the previous courageous conversations with my colleagues were lingering in my mind and tugging at my heart.

Although my colleague's professional practices were not being investigated, both knew they felt compromised by stress and felt stuck as to how to fix the problem. Today, they continue to work as licensed SUD treatment providers. One is in a different position with a different employer. The other made significant changes including reducing their work hours. Both are much happier with their work-life balance.

The primary purpose and function of Licensing Boards is to protect the public from harm by regulating professional practices. All complaints regarding the practice of a licensed professional are reviewed. Those complaints not dismissed due to lack of evidence continue through a process that may or may not result in termination of the license to practice or various levels of sanctions on the license to practice. In New Hampshire, the Office of Professional Licensing and Credentialing (OPLC) is where all the regulating Boards are located. Board activity including results of investigations can be viewed on their website: www.oplc.nh.gov/.

Resilience: The Biology of Stress and the Science of Hope

Around this same time, I had seen the 2016 documentary film James Redford produced and directed based on the findings of the 1997 Adverse Childhood Experiences Study (ACES). The name of the film says it all regarding its message and I have borrowed it to use as the title for the second part of this book—Resilience: The Biology of Stress and the Science of Hope.

Promoting Health Through Happiness

The Bounce Back Project is a unique collaborative of physicians, nurses, hospital leaders, staff, and community partners in Wright County, Minnesota, who have come together for a single purpose—to impact the lives of individuals, communities, and organizations by promoting health through happiness.

This definition of resilience is posted on their website: **Resilience is our ability to bounce back** from the stressors of life. It is not about avoiding the stress, but learning to thrive within the stress, and building more effective coping skills that we can use to deal with the stressful situations. www.bouncebackproject.org/

Dr. Nadine Burke Harris, a pediatrician in San Francisco, is featured in the film at practice in her office with her patients and their families. She is intervening early with her young patients who are at greater risk for diabetes and asthma as well as learning and behavior problems. The outcomes of her care show reduction in the risks predicted by the ACE Study, thus Science of Hope in the subtitle of the film.

Find more information about Dr. Burke Harris and the ACES Quiz in the Resource section of the Action Guide Workbook.

This documentary translates the complexities revealed by the ACE Study. The outcomes of this study are the first empirically validated large-scale study in the U.S. confirming the causal relationship between early childhood hardships and trauma and chronic disease such as diabetes and cardiovascular disease.

The original investigators who created the study are interviewed. You will find multiple resources generated by this study and the original report on the Center for Disease Control website and in the Resource section of the Action Guide Workbook.

The interviews in Redford's documentary validate how research, data, and science can be leveraged as instruments of hope. Leveraging evidence-based research as an instrument of hope is made possible through practical applications that are relevant to the patient or client. The positive outcomes from empowering personal choices reduce the negative consequences identified by the ACE study.

When our patients and clients "get it" as in "how" to integrate and use these applications in their lives, they are empowered to transform life's hard knocks and trauma into resilient building opportunities.

The CDC-Kaiser Permanente Adverse Childhood Experiences (ACE) Study

is one of the largest investigations of childhood abuse and neglect and household challenges and later-life health and well-being. It identified stress as a causal factor of chronic disease and therefore reduced mortality.

The original ACE Study was conducted at Kaiser Permanente from 1995 to 1997 with two waves of data collection. Over 17,000 Health Maintenance Organization members from Southern California receiving physical exams completed confidential surveys regarding their childhood experiences and current health status and behaviors.

Taken from the Center for Disease Control website.

Okay, back to the Ethics training. By now, I am on the edge of my seat waiting for the presentation to talk about ethical standards of practice or reference to the codes of ethics we are sworn to follow regarding self-care or impaired practice prevention (NAADAC). The material presented was incredibly relevant and valuable. But I was looking for something specific, and at that point I had not yet articulated it other than a gut feeling.

During a break, I approached the attorney and commented on the code of ethics for SUD treatment providers including language identifying self-care and self-monitoring as methods for preventing impaired practice.

My initial question for the attorney leading the training was, "How many of your cases involve impaired practice?" However, as I listened to her response, the question I needed to ask became clear:

Is there a measuring stick for identifying when impaired practice becomes an ethical violation?

We talked through the entire break and the room filled up with attendees before we stopped. She handed me a crinkled-up brochure and said, "You and Sally need to get together; call her."

The attorney was right. Since connecting with Sally, she has been and continues to be a tremendous resource and source of inspiration. In fact, later that year, she was one of my primary sources when I teamed up with the Grafton County Prosecutor Lara Saffo to co-facilitate an Ethics training for the New Hampshire Association for Mental Health Counselors on the topic of treating patients with SUD.

Find Lara Saffo's contribution to the Turning Point Stories in the Transcripts.

Dr. Sally Garhart, MD is the Medical Director of the non-profit New Hampshire Professionals Health Program (NHPHP). Their team has created a flagship program providing services and advocating for the well-being and recovery of New Hampshirehealth care professionals.

She is one of original contributors to what became the North Country Task Force on Improving Opioid Treatment Outcomes by Focusing on Provider Resilience and Well-Being. Dr. Garhart is dedicated to serving our healthcare colleagues in times of need and advocating for more effective and compassionate means for doing this while also remaining true to our first call of duty to do no harm.

From this point forward, The North Country Task Force on Improving Opioid Treatment Outcomes by Focusing on Provider Well-Being and Resilience will be referred to as the North Country Task Force throughout the text.

NHPHP provides professional services when determination of a complaint about a healthcare provider includes further evaluation to determine if a medical condition might have contributed to impaired practice as well as other services. This is a simple description of a more complex system and is beyond the scope of this book. However, I have included mention of NHPHP because they offer part of the solution to the burnout dilemma for New Hampshire's healthcare workforce.

Encouraging the Well-Being and Recovery of NH Health Care Professionals through Compassion, Education, Advocacy, Hope.

New Hampshire Professional Health Program

Dr. Garhart shares the timeline of her career and the turning points influencing her decision to join NHPHP as their Medical Director. Her story establishes the foundation for the courageous conversations to follow.

Find her contribution to the Turning Point Stories and update in the Transcripts.

Dr. Garhart shares in her interview experiences in her career that lead her to full-time advocacy for healthcare professional well-being. *As an internal medicine resident at University of Massachusetts Medical Center in Worcester, I got called by the Intensive Care Unit nurses when an obviously impaired nurse anesthetist was unable to extubate a patient which is an exceedingly easy procedure. I calmed him down, did the procedure, and then escorted him to the ER where a tox screen showed 4 injected, diverted substances; I hope that he was sent for treatment and not just fired. A surgical intern committed suicide prompting my medicine intern who was acting very withdrawn to ask me about the suicide rate of our program which was a terrifying question but I calmly told him zero, assigned him more work then went to the chief resident for help. The intern went to treatment and changed fields to something less depressing. That same year, an anesthesia resident died of an overdose on call.*

I learned that the practice of medicine was dangerous and could be lethal due to substance abuse and/or mental health issues. At that point, I was focused on primary care as a career and knew that I needed more communication skills to help patients change habits that were slowly killing them so I rotated through Behavioral Medicine as an elective with a goal of learning smoking cessation skills. There I met Jon Kabat Zinn, PhD before he was famous, seeing consults and attending his groups for chronic pain patients that included meditation and yoga. I witnessed chronically ill patients regain hope and control over disease. Since then I have tried to teach patients and now healthcare professionals how to care for themselves and have consciously practiced mindfulness daily since 1984.

Dr. Garhart also has a knack for distilling down complicated statistical information into a simple one liner like the 80/20 rule. She says this knack developed over the years she has been delivering "elevator statements" during public comments at legislative hearings. In New Hampshire, delivering your message and your request in two minutes or less is the norm at legislative hearings.

The precious 20% is my one liner. The precious 20% is what I call "the punchline" of two sources for what Dr. Garhart calls the 80/20 rule. The 80% is the rest of our workload that includes the administrative tasks required to fulfill practice obligations boiling down to the financial bottom line of fiscal responsibility.

The American Psychological Association (APA) invested significant effort identifying a means for determining impaired practice. I see this continuum as another contributing reference for the measuring stick, I inquired about with the attorney leading the prior mentioned ethics training. The APA describes impairment in terms of a continuum involving stress-distress-impairment-improper behavior.

It is in the nature of this professional work that individuals may develop personal difficulties that impede or impair their personal and professional functioning (O'Connor).

- *Impairment,…refers to "…impairment of ability to practice according to acceptable and prevailing standards of care" (Ohio Administrative Code.)*
- *Impairment therefore refers to circumstances where professional ability is compromised and may negatively impact the delivery of professional services by the psychologist.*

- *Impairment, while heightening the risk for ethical violations, does not infer such violations.*

For myself, and with those I am responsible for supervising, I prefer to focus on the 20% precious compassion satisfaction because it marks the spot on the measuring stick of work-life balance where burnout occurs. This is a concrete point of reference in the process of finding solutions. In this case, to improve our strategies for establishing and maintaining our well-being.

I find it more pleasurable and satisfying to pursue something desirable than avoiding something dreadful. I think of this as the power of positivity. Focusing on the incentive as "a carrot" rather than being frightened by "a big stick".

The question is:
HOW do we achieve and maintain this precious
20% of compassion satisfaction?

I believe Dr. Beth Stamm, PhD, offers the most relevant information for defining the precious 20%. Dr. Stamm developed the Professional Quality of Life (ProQOL) self-score measure in 1995. It is the most used measure of the negative and positive effects of helping others and has been translated in twenty-six languages. You will find a comprehensive bibliography of documents specifically using the ProQOL measure by visiting www.proqol.org.

Compassion Satisfaction defined.

Compassion satisfaction is about the pleasure you derive from being able to do your work. For example, you may feel like it is a pleasure to help others through what you do at work. You may feel positively about your colleagues or your ability to contribute to the work setting or even the greater good of society through your work with people who need care. Compassion Fatigue is the opposite of compassion satisfaction. Fatigue is the negative aspect of helping those who experience traumatic stress and suffering and is the opposite of compassion satisfaction ("Professional Quality of Life").

In the simplest terms, Compassion Satisfaction, (CS) and Compassion Fatigue (CF) can be thought of in simple terms as the positive aspects of helping or the "Good Stuff" (CS) and the negative aspects of helping, that is the "Bad Stuff" (CF) associated with our work as helpers.

Thinking in terms of the good things and bad things associated with helping others who experience suffering is not a theory. Research over the past 30 years has helped clarify the theory of Compassion Satisfaction and Compassion Fatigue and create a data informed theoretical model of (CS-CF Model).

Professional Quality of Life.

According to the CS-CF Model, **Compassion Satisfaction and Compassion Fatigue** are two aspects of Professional Quality of Life. They encompass the positive (Compassion Satisfaction) and the negative (Compassion Fatigue) parts of helping others who have experienced suffering. Compassion fatigue breaks into two parts. The first part concerns things like exhaustion, frustration, anger, and depression typical of burnout. Secondary Traumatic Stress is a negative feeling driven by fear and work-related trauma and can include feeling preoccupied with or having disturbing dreams with the negative details from the history of our clients

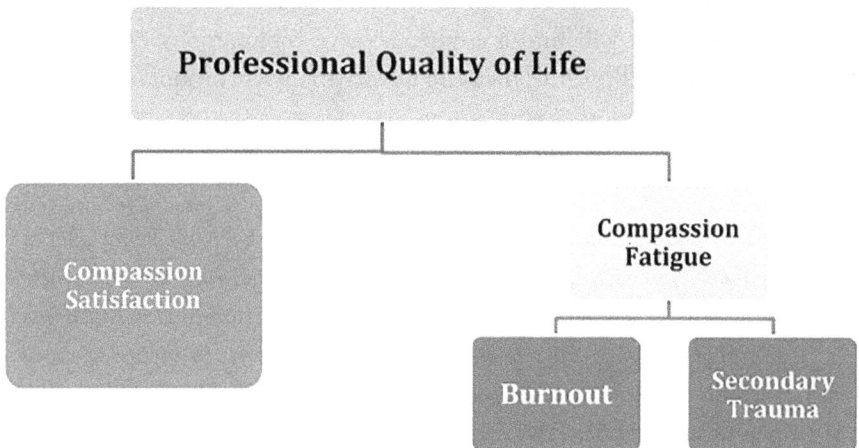

Illustration Slide from the proqol.com resources

Regarding trauma. It is important to remember that some trauma at work can be direct (primary) trauma. In other cases, work-related trauma is a combination of both primary and secondary trauma. If working with others' suffering changes you so deeply in negative ways that your understanding of yourself changes, this is vicarious traumatization. Learning from and understanding vicarious traumatization can lead one to vicarious transformation. More detailed information can be found in the ProQOL Manual (Stamm, 2010) and on the ProQOL website.

Invitation for Reflection and Action

What was your reaction to learning about the 80/20 rule?

Do you believe 20% meaningful and productive work is enough for you to avoid burnout?

How do you define meaningful and productive work in your job responsibilities?

Where do you experience this in your work and how often?

Let all this settle in.

If you have access to being outdoors, consider taking a short walk or stand up if you have been sitting or simply pay attention to what your mind and body is calling for right now and respond.

Out of the numerous available definitions and interpretations of work-life balance, I found Jim Bird's description most in alignment with what I know to be true for myself as well as for many of my colleagues. Jim Bird is the founder of WorkLifeBalance.com and recognized internationally as a leading work-life balance company. The description posted on their website focuses on achievement and enjoyment as the core foundation within four areas of life: work, family, friends, and self.

Work-Life Balance Defined

Let us first define what work-life balance *is not*.

Work-Life Balance *does not mean an equal balance*. Trying to schedule an equal number of hours for each of your various work and personal activities is usually unrewarding and unrealistic. Life is and should be more fluid than that.

Your best individual work-life balance will vary over time, often daily. The right balance for you today will probably be different for you tomorrow. The right balance for you when you are single will be different when you marry, or if you have children, when you start a new career versus when you are nearing retirement.

There is no perfect "one-size fits all" balance you should be striving for. The best work-life balance is different for each of us because we all have different priorities and different lives.

www.WorkLifeBalance.com

Achievement and enjoyment are identified as the core foundation within four areas of life: work, family, friends, and self in Jim Bird's definition for work-life balance. The precious 20% of compassion satisfaction is similar in that for healthcare and behavioral health direct service providers, achievement is also defined as meaningful and purposeful work has been done. Knowing our work is making a positive difference is the achievement.

CHAPTER ONE SUMMARY

In this chapter, the concepts discussed in this book for defining and addressing the burnout dilemma are presented. According to the World Health Organization, **burnout** is an occupational phenomenon due to unsuccessful managed chronic workplace stressors and characterized by three criteria: feelings of energy depletion, increased mental distancing from one's job, and cynicism or reduced professional efficacy. **Work-life balance** is identified as being unique to each person and includes four areas of life: work, family, friends, and self with achievement and enjoyment at the core of each. The **80/20**

ratio gives us a concrete reference for defining our **precious 20% compassion satisfaction.** Hopeful outcomes are also reviewed from the application of preventive measures to reduce risks of illness and chronic disease linked to adverse childhood experiences as demonstrated by the ACE Study.

CHAPTER ONE KEY POINTS

Burnout is characterized by:

Feelings of energy depletion or exhaustion.

Increased mental distancing from one's job, or feelings of negativism or cynicism related to one's job, and reduced professional efficacy.

ACE Study validates the causal relationship between early childhood adverse experiences and the onset of chronic disease and early onset of mortality.

Primary Care and Pediatricians are applying preventive care to reduce the risks caused by adverse childhood experiences of their patients. See the documentary Resilience: The Biology of Stress and the The Science of Hope.

Self-care and self-monitoring are mentioned in three of the nine Principles of the National Association for Alcohol and Drug Abuse Counselors Code of Ethics: III. Professional Responsibility and Workplace Standards, VII. Supervision and Consultation, VIII. Resolving Ethical Concerns (NAADAC).

Impaired practice is to be expected and does not necessarily mean ethical violation.

The 80/20 rule means 80% Administrative responsibilities and at least 20% meaningful and productive patient to provider interaction.

Work-life balance is unique to each person and includes four areas of life: work, family, friends, and self with achievement and enjoyment at the core of each.

Compassion satisfaction is an outcome of achieving a sense of purpose and meaning in your work helping others and finding enjoyment in that process.

Precious 20% compassion satisfaction is the minimum necessary to keep burnout at bay in our work-life balance.

How the Problem Came to Be

> **"Insanity is doing the same thing over and over again and expecting different results."**
>
> *Albert Einstein*
>
> Quote contribution by Dr. Sally Garhart, MD
> Medical Director of the New Hampshire Professionals Health Program
> Go to the Turning Point Stories & Interview Transcripts to find Dr. Garhart's full story.

CRISIS IS OPPORTUNITY

CHAPTER TWO PREVIEW

In this chapter my lived experience planning to end my life by suicide and Panda's role (Registered Therapy Dog) as an interventionist is woven with relevant research to describe how this crisis became an opportunity. As part of my recovery plan, my sister Cynthia Thomas left Virginia to live with me in New Hampshire. Seeing my work-life balance through her eyes combined with insights from her career in public health and chronic disease management added to our shared family history infused a healing process for both of us we never expected.

As a therapist, a clinical supervisor, as a person in long-term recovery, a mother, daughter, friend, neighbor, and colleague, I wanted to find a way to speak to the relevant data and how to be transparent with my crisis experience. I knew this story needed to be delivered in a way to inform future SUD workforce development. Effectively building a resilient workforce means honestly addressing the challenges our workers are facing on the frontline and how this impacts the quality of care being delivered.

In Our Own Voice training sponsored by the National Alliance for Mental Illness (NAMI) provided me with a template for how to craft and deliver such a story. The timing was right for a provider needs assessment and the outcomes fueled momentum that led to eleven colleagues joining me in 2018 to deliver their turning point stories as testimony to what they are doing to maintain their own precious 20% compassion satisfaction.

In Our Own Voice

Eleven colleagues crafted two to three-minute individual Turning Point stories as part of the presentation on Clinician Well-Being for Improved Treatment Outcomes. We modeled our format similarly to the NAMI In Our Own Voice format for telling our story focused on what happened, what helped, and what next ("NAMI").

Find many of these Turning Point stories in the Interview Transcripts.

One of the outcomes of this presentation launched The North Country Task Force on Improving Opioid Treatment Outcomes by Focusing on Provider Well-Being. Every time I write that long title, I smile remembering Tonya Tavares coaching me on the importance of selecting vocabulary to fit grant qualification criteria. She was one of several technical assistance providers who encouraged the development and the work represented in this book. Her role linked the Task Force to a national network and as a result everyone involved not only felt heard but also validated. Isolation due to being in a rural region was no longer perceived as a barrier. This validation strengthened our resolve to continue and helped us to recognize our rural and small community network as our strength rather than a barrier.

Tonya Tavares, MS, CCRP
Assistant Project Director for the Opioid Response Network
STR-TA Technology Transfer Specialist at the Center for Alcohol and
Addictions Studies Brown University New England, Region 1- CT, MA,
ME, NH, RI, VT

Find Tonya's full interview in the Transcripts.

Hindsight is 20/20 in 2020

The events reviewed thus far represent early stages of change in my own work-life balance awareness. Looking back, it is easy for me to see what I did not see at the time. At that point in time, I was in what DiClemente and Prochaska identify in their Stages of Change Model (DiClemente) as pre-contemplation regarding my own well-being and work-life balance. Looking back, I can see how old unhelpful habits crept back into my way of functioning. This contributed to the downward spiral of my overall well-being.

My thoughts were focused outside of myself contemplating the dilemma my two colleagues had presented to me many months prior. The circumstances of my work demanded I remain focused on "what is best for the program". I have always been resilient and expected myself to be able to handle whatever came my way. I was still grieving the loss of my mother and preoccupied with concern for my father's condition plus other normal family life transitions and adjustments. Everything happening in a short period of time pushed me to adopt a bite the bullet, pull up your big girl pants, and keep your nose to the grindstone attitude.

Looking back, I see how my "normal" work ethic code is hard-assed. These expectations of myself, rooted in how I was raised, had worked to my advantage in the past. This multi-generational work ethic code of honor became a rigid, fixed expectation stuck in unrealistic belief and fed this perfect storm. Any ONE of these events is enough stress to justify using sick time, vacation time, or other forms of "paid time off". Everything combined together with my rigid loyalty to my family work ethic legacy became a life-threatening crisis.

Stages of Change Model

The concept of a spiral is intended to reflect that in real life change rarely happens in a straight line but rather in a spiral moving forward while learning from our experience and applying those lessons as we go.

Pre-Contemplation: No intention of changing behavior.

Contemplation: Aware a problem exists but with no commitment to action.

Preparation: Intention on taking action to address the problem.

Action: Active modification of behavior.

Maintenance: Sustained change; new behavior replaces old.

Relapse: Fall back into old patterns of behavior.

Approximately a year after the ethics training described in chapter one, I resigned from my full-time job as Clinical Director of a large SUD Treatment Center. That was early in the spring of 2017. By then, I completely understood what my trusted colleagues were experiencing the prior year. Separately and independent of one another, they confided in me their anguish and sense of helplessness about their work. No longer feeling effective at making a difference and not seeing hope in the future for the circumstances to improve, both of my colleagues wanted to throw in the towel. One was considering giving up their license to practice and going to work at something completely different and unrelated to human services. The other had a plan to end their life by suicide. In less than a year's time, I found myself in their shoes experiencing exactly what I had heard them describe to me.

Up until that time, the challenges I had experienced in my career had been transient and short-term. That made it easier to get through the rough patches because I knew there was light at the end of the tunnel.

This time, I didn't care.
I was too tired to care.

Several years leading up to that point in early spring 2017, our family had lost my mother to cancer, my father was experiencing an unusual medical condition causing him to lose his ability to swallow and later diagnosed as Myasthenia Gravis. Several other significant life transitions combined with my work-related challenges became a perfect storm for my own crisis.

My work-life balance was no longer connected with compassion satisfaction. Several months leading up to the day I planned to end my life, I was functioning robotically. I remember commenting to someone about being "a cog in the machine" in response to their polite greeting of "How are you doing?" I was still eating, sleeping, and tending to my personal hygiene but that was pretty much it. My social life had become non-existent and most importantly, I had stopped seeing my therapist, stopped speaking with my peer collaboration group, stopped practicing nearly all my self-care and recovery-based tools because I was too F*#*g tired to care.

Panda the Therapy Dog

During the three years up to that point, I had trained a new Therapy Dog to become part of my practice. Her name is Panda. About eight years prior to that, I adopted "Harley", an adult mixed breed dog from a colleague who is a psychologist. Harley had become quite popular with his clients. They were no longer able to keep Harley and wanted to find another home where Harley could continue "doing her job". I've had dogs as a pet for practically my entire life and loved the idea of being able to have a dog join me in my office. Harley and I passed the performance test and Harley became Internationally Registered as Therapy Dog in 2007. In anticipation of Harley's retirement, I adopted a young border collie named Panda. She quickly picked up the skills and earned Therapy Dog Registration. She attended nearly every group and individual counseling session I led at the County Jail and at the SUD treatment center.

Panda had been accompanying me every day on the job. She had become to me like what Peter Pan's shadow was to him. You know, sort of like one. But on this day, approximately six weeks after I left my job at the SUD treatment center, I was not thinking about Panda being with me. That is how disengaged and robotic my behavior and thinking had become over the several months leading up to then._

I had not considered Panda being part of my plan for suicide. My plan was to stage my death in such a way that it would appear to have been an accident so my family would receive the pay out on my life insurance policy. My worries about financial responsibilities had become my focal point. I could not see any other solutions for resolving our financial debts.

At the time, I believed this was the solution.

Panda was with me on the day I was going to carry out my plan. But I was not aware of her being with me. That is how robotic and out of touch I was. We were walking together on one of our favorite trails. What she did was not dramatic, but it was unusual. Panda placed herself ahead of me then turned to face me in the herding position she uses when anticipating a game of fetch with a Frisbee. I thought her behavior was odd because we never play Frisbee while walking on trails.

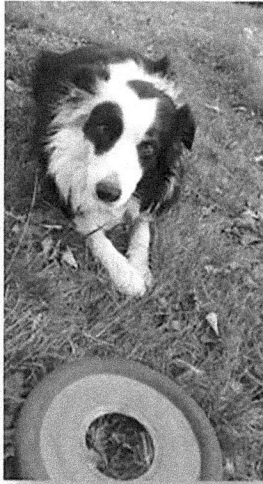

Panda with her favorite Frisbee
Photo taken by Franconia Jones

We returned to my car, where we played fetch in the empty parking lot. When playtime was over, I calmly made arrangements for admission into psychiatric care. I was fortunate to find an opening that same afternoon rather than having to wait several days for a bed to be available at a psychiatric treatment center. Over the many years of helping others enter recovery, I had learned a thing or two about expediting treatment admissions and was able to use this experience to my advantage. Fortunately, Panda was with me and helped me remember to do for myself what I had done for many others.

Later, I recognized I had lost touch with my thirty-something years as a person in long-term recovery from alcohol and cannabis use disorders. Up until that moment, I believed I was okay because I had not relapsed or felt urges or cravings—classic symptoms a relapse is on its way. However, I did think about smoking weed again. The thought was like a fleeting fantasy. But honestly the memory of my last experiences with it, thirty some odd years ago, and how anxious and paranoid it caused me to be, quickly squelched that fleeting thought.

Nevertheless, this was a signal of my distress, and I ignored it because I believed I could tough it out.

Looking back, it is easy for me to see how the illogical thinking I developed as a young person was a product of the maladaptive survival thinking I had grown to rely on prior to developing a substance use disorder. I'm referring to the loyal unspoken code of honor embedded into my work ethic.

This thinking includes unrealistic and negative self-talk like, suck it up buttercup, get a grip, quit your bellyaching, you've been through worse than this, pull yourself together!

Although I had no prior history of major depression or suicidal thoughts, ending my life by suicide felt rational and logical.

At the time, I did not think of it as suicide but rather as a solution to end what felt like impossible circumstances.

My old belief system that defined my hard-ass work ethic included never relying on anyone for help and, oddly enough, became a comfort because of its familiarity despite it being part of a life I had left behind thirty years ago. I will explain more about this in part two, the Biology of Stress and the Science of Hope.

Find my early recovery story in Sue Thistle's 2020 Bestseller,

"Chem-Free Sobriety: 101 Trailblazers share wisdom and insight about their natural recovery from substance use disorders".

Also find an updated live recorded version called "Valuing Self-Care" posted on **the Granite State News Collaborative YouTube channel in Community Engagement.**

The ripple effect of our workforce shortage meant an increase in visits related to the treatment of substance use disorders at primary care offices, in schools and classrooms, interactions with public safety, and in the workplace.

Employee Assistance Program referrals from the surrounding employers tripled in my part-time private practice. All reported work-life balance challenges and feelings of burnout due to shortages of staff and the shortage of services to address our community's need for SUD treatment.

After seeing many of the same people come and go through the revolving door of treatment, seeing no evidence of change, and seeing a steady reduction of resources while the need for treatment continued growing, I began to feel ineffective at my job. My compassion satisfaction meter began to drop rapidly.

While in treatment at the psychiatric hospital, I felt a weird sort of relief to speak out loud about all of this with others. I could see they understood how it is possible to believe illogical thinking offered the best solution, which meant, to me, permanently eliminating myself from the equation.

I thought I would feel ashamed or embarrassed because I didn't "keep to my code of honor".

Panda's sweet unconditional intervention cleansed me of that. Really. Her precious devoted loyalty and pure joy playing Frisbee immediately brought me back into the reality of that tragic thinking.

During my four-day hospital stay, my description of work-life imbalance was affirmed as a shared reality and especially from the staff. I began to see, feel, and think more clearly. As part of my discharge plan, I knew I needed to move this conversation into a public forum. I wanted to engage in meaningful and productive discussions about how work culture norms that promote self-sacrifice and feeding an unhealthy work-life balance, contributes to burn-out, and ultimately erodes our first duty as helpers, which is to do no harm.

My sister, Cindi, and I had been talking with each other on the telephone almost daily. The medical issues with both of our parents had caused me and both of my sisters to be in touch with one another more frequently. Because of Cindi's familiarity with hospital procedures, our family relies on her to translate and explain whatever the medical providers recommend and so on. I was in the Emergency Room of the hospital I admitted myself to when she called. She was shocked when I told her where I was and why I was there. That is how good I was at hiding the truth about how I was feeling. She had no idea I had been planning to end my life by suicide.

Turns out, research about suicide shows it is not uncommon for people who die by suicide do not leave notes or display warning signs.

Suicide often not preceded by warnings

"Many people never let on what they are feeling or planning. The paradox is that the people who are most intent on committing suicide know that they have to keep their plans to themselves if they are to carry out the act," says Dr. Miller. "Thus, the people most in need of help may be the toughest to save"(Skerrett).

Sistah Power

I am seven and nine years younger than my two sisters. As it is with most adult siblings, our love for one another has always felt deep and binding, despite our episodes of not seeing eye-to-eye, our time together as adults has been limited to holidays and special occasions.

As it is with families growing up and getting older, get-togethers dwindle down to weddings or funerals. The last time the three of us were together was during the last months of our mother's life in 2015. Kathryn (I've always called her Kathy), my oldest sister shouldered the role of power of attorney for Mom and managed practically every business detail there was to deal with before and after Mom died. Out of the three of us, Kathy has always had the head for business.

During that period of time in 2015, our mother's death brought us together, obviously. There was something different about this togetherness other than shared grief. We were sitting on the back porch sorting through our parents' hope chest. Consciously or subconsciously, the hope chest had been left to one of the last things we did together to prepare for the sale of her home. While sorting through decades of memories, we found a collection of photos, cards, and baby clothing we had never seen. These items were from Kathryn's birth, mom and dad's high school graduations, and good wishes for their marriage.

Kathryn is the first born of the three of us and the story we knew about this was Mom and Dad married before their high school graduation. For us, and especially for Kathyrn, the vibe of that story carried a heaviness to it. Our mom downplayed the story. It always felt mysterious and because we grew up in southwest Virginia during the 1950s and '60s, well, we assumed the political and religious culture of that time must have cast shame into that story. So, we left it alone.

We must have read nearly one hundred hand written notes and cards of good wishes, congratulations, and other blessings and comments filled with hope. The photos with this archive of memories captured these precious and delightful moments. The three of us witnessed a beautiful period of time in our parents' lives without anyone else's interpretation. Those pictures really did speak a thousand words.

In that moment the three of us recognized something had shifted. Words weren't needed. The vibe was enough. A feeling of peace and contentment shared between us. Since then we use the term **Sistah Power** when we're sharing that vibe.

Cindi's lifetime career in public health leadership and chronic disease management combined with our shared life experiences generated new wind for my sails and helped me see my path moving forward. Even though I was also receiving outpatient therapy and maintaining my medical appointments with my doctor, having my sister with me was by far my best medicine. Not having to explain where certain ways of thinking or behaving came from because we shared much of the same gave me a sense of safety and protection I really needed at that time—something, in my subjective opinion, a therapist, a doctor, group therapy, or a self-help group can't do unless that other person has shared their life story that also validates the experience.

> To effectively raise awareness
> about risks to patient care and safety
> due to worker fatigue and burnout,
>
> **I needed relevant validating data**
> other than my own subjective experience.

Being able to talk freely as part of the natural course of the day was especially helpful. Although she had her work schedule and I had my own schedule, sharing the same living space, sharing meals together, and having free time together made it easier for me to process my experience and sort out my next steps. She joined me in several of my therapy sessions and conference calls with my husband who was working full-time on the west coast at the time.

Not being alone in my house all the time was a key factor that expedited my healing. Several weeks after my return home, I knew I did not want to return to full-time work managing a SUD treatment center. Throughout my career I have maintained a small private practice and returning to work in that setting felt like the right next move.

Peer Collaboration. Cindi joined me in my small peer collaboration group. This group meets once a month for two hours. It is an accountability measure required for license retention for SUD and mental health clinicians in New Hampshire. My peer collaboration group was the first public place I disclosed my recent crisis. After several months of processing together, we were unanimous about speaking up together about the importance for work culture norms to engage proactive employment practices supporting worker well-being.

With encouragement from my sisters, family, and colleagues, I regained confidence and relaxed into trusting myself again. Cindi's expertise in public health made the next steps easier. The time came when I recognized it was time for me to step up and start walking my talk beyond my own backyard. Cindi helped me push through my insecurities with politicking. The timing was good. The North Country Region Representative seat on the Board of Directors of the New Hampshire Association for Drug and Alcohol Counselors (NHADACA) was vacant. With my sister's encouragement, I responded to the call for volunteers from the Board of Directors and submitted my bio and statement of intent. No one else was on the ballot for the North Country Region Representative and so my term as North Country Region Representative began.

Cindi coached me through using the free version of SurveyMonkey to develop and tabulate a Provider Needs Assessment based on the Professional Quality of Life measure discussed in chapter one.

We coordinated with the local community health agencies to get it distributed. We distributed it to two-hundred people and received a 17% response rate. For the North Country and two weeks before Christmas, we thought this was darned good. And, no, Christmastime was not the intended distribution time.

However, responses indicated people were ready to start talking about work-life balance.

2018 North Country Provider Needs Assessment outcomes

96% of respondents reported at risk of burnout
Less than 45% reported receiving clinical supervision, and
are NOT talking
about these symptoms
because of fear they would lose their job.

**Let that sink in;
nearly half the respondents
did not mention burnout symptoms during supervision
because they feared job loss.**

Invitation for Reflection and Action

Are you currently experiencing joy or satisfaction in your personal or professional life?

List examples of the thoughts, actions or behavior, your emotion when you are experiencing joy or satisfaction:

Do you experience personal satisfaction differently from how you experience professional satisfaction?

What can you do to increase experiencing joy or satisfaction in your personal and/or professional life?

Your SMART goals: **S**pecific
$\qquad\qquad$ **M**easurable
$\qquad\qquad$ **A**chievable
$\qquad\qquad$ **R**elevant
$\qquad\qquad$ **T**ime Bound

The data collected from this regional provider needs assessment gave us the validation needed to carry this small grassroots momentum of courageous conversations into a larger audience. I also accepted the position of Chairperson for the NHADACA Ethics Committee which had been inactive for several years. After researching the activity and history of this committee and consulting with the National Association for Alcohol and Drug Addiction Counselors (NAADAC), I developed a proposal to update the scope of this committee to be in more alignment with the current needs of our SUD workforce in New Hampshire.

Rebecca Libby, School Counselor in New Hampshire describes in her 2018 Turning Point story how the death of a colleague at work impacted her and began her journey of commitment to self-care.

__A major turning point for me__ as a school counselor was when a colleague died at work. Martha had been working 1:1 with a student with a traumatic brain injury when she unexpectedly died of a heart attack at school. I was one of the first to respond to the emergency. During the time of Martha's death, I worked with our emergency management team to provide treatment. I was with Martha's *sister and Maura when the doctor confirmed that she had died. I do not remember how I got home that afternoon; I cried the whole way. I returned to work the next day ready to take care of the staff and students needing support. A colleague looked at me and said, "You don't always have to be so strong."*

My colleague was right. It's so easy to start our workday and just go full speed ahead. Before we know it, the day is over, and we have not taken a lunch break or even had a second to run to the restroom. In our profession we cannot run at this speed and think we are invincible.

Eventually we will run out of steam.

The research I had been doing on provider well-being led me to discover a parallel process occurring across the nation. The National Academy of Medicine (NAM) announced in 2017 their Call to Action for Clinician Well Being (*National Academy of Medicine*). This is yet another outcome initiated by the 1999 report *To Err is Human* mentioned in chapter one.

The timing was right. In the fall of 2018, several colleagues joined Cindi and I at the 26th Annual New England School of Best Practices in Addiction Treatment. In a six-hour workshop, we shared our lived experiences described as Turning Point Stories with approximately thirty people. This combined with the data collected from the Provider Needs Assessment and the research made available from the NAM Action Collaborative validated what had been unspoken for many of the participants.

Participants commented the workshop felt it was like a coming out experience.

> Combining authentic lived experience
> with relevant data and research
> became an effective platform for introducing the opportunity for others
> to enter courageous conversations.
>
> Find many of the Turning Point Stories with the Interview Transcripts.

As a result of this workshop, we were introduced to the Opioid Response Network. Through their Technical Assistance, the **North Country Task Force** for **Improving Opioid Treatment Outcomes by Focusing on Provider Well-Being and Resilience was established**. This book is a product of that work and evidence of how a small grassroots movement can become part of a national movement.

The Task Force aligned its goals with this national initiative and within eighteen months our progress enabled the workgroups to begin working autonomously. After many months of educating the Board of Directors about NAM's initiative, NHADACA became the first New Hampshire Networking Organization and published a Commitment Statement for Clinician Well-Being.

The following year, Dr. Art Hengerer, MD, co-chair of the NAM Action Collaborative on Clinician Well-Being delivered the keynote presentation at the 2019 New Hampshire Annual Behavioral Health Conference held in Manchester. Additionally, as a Network Organization, NHADACA was able to host the NAM Action Collaborative Expression of Clinician Well-Being. This is a traveling art exhibit of original pieces of art produced by clinicians across the country expressing their journey into clinician well-being ("Expressions").

Having my sister with me while I was reconnecting with my sense of place in my work-life balance gave me the opportunity to see myself through her eyes. Her love for working in the soil and in my gardens that had gone neglected during my too tired to care period encouraged me. Watching her enjoy the pleasure of resurrecting an overgrown and hidden blueberry patch invited me to revisit doing something I never imagined abandoning. We started with several forty year or so bushes I transplanted from a friend's yard. That summer not only did we resurrect nearly all my perennial, vegetable, and blueberry gardens, I also reclaimed my sense of place with my life.

Reclaiming my sense of place at my home,
in my gardens and on the land, with my family,
and in my practice is how I began
rebuilding my precious *compassion satisfaction* in
my work-life balance.

The concept of sense of place has been used in terms of architectural and landscape design as well as community development and formally referred to as place attachments (Stedman).

The Place Attachment theory primarily focuses on the emotional attachment to places or things and how this influences our choices and preferences for where to live, work, visit, etc. During my too tired to care period, I lost touch with that and although I am profoundly connected to my home and the land around our home, I also recognize another sense of place with my work that doesn't seem to be connected to a place or thing but rather to a feeling. The best way I can describe this feeling is with familiar slang words or phrases like "being in the zone" and "the sweet spot". I think each of us have our own recipe of these things and this recipe is the superhighway to compassion satisfaction. The second part of the book will review some of the neurobiological explanations for this.

I will close this chapter with an introduction to the North Country. Early in my adult life, I learned the meaning of "absence makes the heart grow fonder" when I left the east coast to live in Colorado. During that time in my life, I traveled as much as I could and discovered the awesomeness of geographic diversity in this country. Although I appreciate these differences, I learned my preference is for the habitat, climate, and culture of the Appalachian Mountains. The Appalachian Mountains is where I feel the most at home.

The North Country in New Hampshire is the geographic region north of the White Mountains. This section of the Appalachian Mountain Range is considered the most rugged stretch of the 2,190-mile Appalachian Trail extending from the state of Georgia to Maine. The North Country is where my husband and I raised our family and where most of my career has been.

New Hampshire is the fifth smallest state by square miles and the tenth least populous U.S. state ("QuickFacts").

Probably the best description of the North Country that continues to be used today would be from former NH *Governor Sherman Adams who is credited with establishing "north of the Notches." That would be north of Franconia Notch, Crawford Notch, and Pinkham Notch, all in the beautiful White Mountains and Presidential Range to the south. This range of mountains is part of the Appalachian Mountain range stretching from Georgia to Maine. The most southern tip of the 2,190-mile Appalachian Trail starts at Springer Mountain, Georgia and the northern end at Mount Katahdin in Maine.

*White House Chief of Staff (1953–1958), Governor of New Hampshire (1949–1953)

My family roots go back to northern Wales, Scotland, Ireland, England and Germany. While living in Colorado, I grew "homesick" for cloudy and rainy days. While in undergraduate school, I studied abroad in London and Switzerland. While there, I explored Wales and Scotland. Although it was the first time for me to set foot on that land, I felt right at home because of the similarities of the land, climate, and people with the Blue Ridge Mountains of the Appalachia in southwestern Virginia where I was born and raised.

New Hampshire is the fifth smallest state in the U.S. and forests occupy eighty one percent of New Hampshire's land (NH Division of Forests and Lands). I think it is amazing to imagine the fifth smallest state in the U.S. is also the second most forested. The North Country of New Hampshire occupies one third of the entire state and is the least populated area in the state. www.en.wikipedia.org/wiki/New_Hampshire

Hiking in the White Mountains will take you above the treeline. This is spectacular if you like to hike. The foliage and plant life found above treeline is like that in the permafrost region of northwestern Alaska. I had the pleasure of experiencing this during the year we lived in Nome and that is a whole different story for another time in a different book. In New Hampshire, the White Mountains are called "white" because they often have snow on them when nothing else around has snow.

Mount Washington is the highest peak of the White Mountains at elevation 6,288 feet. It is said to be the home to the world's worst weather and the most prominent topographically mountain east of the Mississippi River. To the surprise of many, Mount Washington is not the highest mountain on the east coast. It is 395 feet shorter than Mount Mitchell nineteen miles northeast of Asheville, North Carolina.

The Appalachian Mountains are where me and my husband grew up. Barry is from Nashville, Tennessee and I from Radford, Virginia. We met while attending East Tennessee State University in Johnson City. Right out of college, we began working for the North Carolina Outward Bound School at the Table Rock Mountain Base. He was a Rock-Climbing Instructor and I was a Field Instructor.

Over the course of our lifetime, we have hiked all the 4,000 footers and much of the 2,193-mile Appalachian Trail excluding the sections between the southern end of New England and northern Virginia. When our kids were young, we enjoyed staying in the Appalachian Mountain Club (AMC) Huts. The AMC Hut system is a great way to introduce young children to multiple day hiking along the Presidential Range of mountains.

Turns out we have a knack for working with what was called at that time adjudicated youth; more affectionately referred to as "hoods in the woods". This work took us to New Hampshire as Outward Bound Field Instructors with the Hurricane Island Outward Bound School. A partnership had been forged with Beech Hill Hospital in Dublin, New Hampshire, for establishing a wilderness-based substance use disorder treatment program for youth.

This was my first exposure to the 12-Step self-help program of Alcoholics Anonymous.

Although close friends, some family members, and my husband (at that time my "significant other") had tried talking with me about their concerns for my drinking, I did not see what they were talking about. I fit the category of what some call a high functioning alcoholic. I never had any legal trouble because of drinking, never injured myself, maintained a high-honors grade average, worked two jobs while in school full-time, and never showed up to class or work under the influence. From my point of view, they did not know what they were talking about. **Unfortunately, I could not see that they did.**

The thirty-two-day wilderness treatment model used at the time included a four-member field team of two licensed clinicians and two Outward Bound instructors. Therapeutic psychoeducation modules were delivered daily by the clinical staff. Much of the material was 12-step based and we would attend onsite A.A. meetings in town during resupply. Many of these meetings were in Littleton, the neighboring town where we live now in Bethlehem. I felt drawn to the discussions and started attending A.A. meetings on my own and for myself. Once I found an A.A. Sponsor, I started working through the twelve steps.

The structure of the program gave me what I needed to see what I had not recognized. The one-on-one Sponsor relationship was exactly what I needed to begin integrating the principles of living in recovery. Today, I recognize many roads and pathways of recovery beyond the 12-step program and continue to learn from each person I encounter in my practice and in my work.

Substance Use Disorders (SUD) are a chronic disease. Simply put, this means the symptoms will get worse if untreated and will eventually contribute to or be the cause of death. The Stages of Change model, mentioned earlier, identifies the last step in the process as "relapse". I prefer to use the word recurrence and a forward spiraling line to illustrate the idea of how recovery works. My recent crisis story is an example of how it is possible for someone in recovery from a substance use disorder to relapse or to have a recurrence with old unproductive unhealthy habits and still move forward. In my case, my relapse was not with substances but rather with the recurrence of maladaptive and illogical thinking developed prior to misuse of substances. The opportunity to learn something new or to see something familiar in a new way is always there. It's a matter of getting out of our way to see it.

CHAPTER TWO SUMMARY

Crisis can be an opportunity. Courageous conversations help to break the cycle of doing or thinking the same thing repeatedly and expecting different results. Trusted relationships help us grow our courage to have difficult conversations. Speaking honestly and in a way others can relate is an important step toward reducing the silence that keeps us isolated from opportunities for change. Isolation can often lead to crisis and unnecessary harm or loss. Change is a developmental process and it is helpful to meet people where they are in the change continuum to connect with them in a way that builds trust.

In Our Own Voice program developed by the National Alliance for Mental Illness provides a tested and proven method for preparing ourselves to share courageous conversations. The process of engaged courageous conversations also builds a sense of place for experiencing safety and it is in these spaces the precious 20% begins and is nurtured.

CHAPTER TWO KEY POINTS

The In Our Own Voice Program is part of the National Alliance for Mental Illness and is designed to empower recovery, increase awareness, and reduce stigma associated with mental illness through positive stories about what happened, what helped, and what next.

The Stages of Change are Pre-contemplation, Contemplation, Planning, Action, Maintenance, and Recurrence.

Peer Collaboration and Clinical Supervision are risk management mechanisms to protect patient care and safety

Courageous conversations involve truth speaking from a sense of place.

Family can also be defined as not blood kin but the people we feel unconditional acceptance and safety with

---

Impact of the Problem

> **"Necessity is the mother of invention."**
>
> A need or problem encourages creative efforts to meet the
> need or solve the problem. This saying appears in the dialogue
> *Republic*, by the ancient Greek philosopher Plato.

OCCUPATIONAL PHENOMENON
CHAPTER THREE PREVIEW

This chapter explores work ethic as a cultural factor in the burnout dilemma. The World Health Organization's definition of burnout as an occupational phenomenon is examined in terms of identifying boundaries of responsibility for the employer and the worker. Regional issues previously described are linked with development of occupational safety standards and labor law in the United States through recollection from family history to illustrate how need drives demand and demand drives change. Stamm's perspective of "we bring ourselves to work" as previously described in the Professional Quality of Life measure is also used to illustrate how personal family history influences our perception, belief, and attitude about work ethic. The Opioid Misuse Tool opioidmisusetool.norc.org/ is introduced as a resource for researchers, policymakers, journalists, and the general public to create county-level maps illustrating the relationship between community and population demographics and fatal drug overdoses—including opioids—in the United States. Insights derived from this tool can be used to target resources and interventions and inform media coverage related to overdose deaths in the United States. Interviews with New Hampshire citizens involved with addressing these problems through the New Hampshire Recovery Friendly Workplace Initiative, Recovery Support Centers, and Sober Living communities are introduced.

These individuals speak to their perspectives on the impact of this problem and what they are doing to influence positive change.

In May 2019, the World Health Organization (WHO) announced they are updating its definition of burnout in the new version of its handbook of diseases, the *International Classification of Diseases, ICD-11.*

The International Classification of Diseases
book was first published in 1893 to establish a universal method of identifying and categorizing human diseases. Today, it contains around 55,000 unique codes for injuries, diseases, and causes of death. About 70% of the world's health expenditures (USD 3.5 billion) are allocated using ICD for reimbursement and resource allocation.

The new definition calls burnout "an occupational phenomenon" and includes it in a chapter on "factors influencing health status or contact with health services." This definition specifically ties burnout to "chronic workplace stress that has not been successfully managed." WHO does not classify burnout as a medical condition ("WHO Redefines Burnout").

Worker's well-being is of paramount importance to the productivity, competitiveness, and sustainability of enterprises, communities, and national and regional economies. But the issue extends beyond individuals and their families. The impact of our current global pandemic on the United States and world economy has made this painfully clear.

>**Depression and anxiety have a significant economic impact;** the estimated cost to the global economy is USD 1 trillion per year in lost productivity.

>**Estimated that for every USD 1 put into scaled up treatment for common mental disorders, there is a return of USD 4 in improved health and productivity.**

>**An estimated two million people die each year because of occupational accidents** and work-related illnesses or injuries (Burton).

WHO's definition of burnout:
an occupational phenomenon tied to chronic workplace stress
that has not been successfully managed
begs the question,

Who is responsible for managing workplace stress?

Managing workplace stress is a shared responsibility between the employer and the worker.

Every work environment is unique to the professional practice within it. The community meetings held by the North Country Task Force quickly identified this. While everyone can agree burnout is an experience all of us can relate to equally. Addressing how to fix it needs to be done from within the work culture itself. Therefore, five work groups were established to develop action plans based on their unique work culture: HealthCare, Education, Public Safety, Administration/Policy, Commerce.

Invitation for Reflection and Action

If changes or adjustments are necessary to increase the level of joy or satisfaction in your personal and/or professional life, how will you know your plan is working?

List at least three things you see
> hear
> feel

Is there someone who can help you with this plan? How can they help?

Use SMART goals: **S**pecific
> **M**easurable
> **A**ttainable
> **R**easonable
> **T**ime frame

Set a time and day you will contact someone to express your gratitude for their presence in your life and describe something they have done that has encouraged you.

A common denominator revealed by Task Force discussions is that regardless of the work culture or the profession, **Administrative leadership and the workers must work together** in order to get anywhere with establishing, implementing, and maintaining methods and systems to effectively manage the workplace stressors. This seems obvious and certainly can be easier said than done.

Michael Meit, the developer of the Opioid Misuse Tool in the North Country of New Hampshire where I live and work and in response to the Opioid Overdose Epidemic, many of us who work with the public recognized the importance of working across the continuum of care. In 2016, I was still in the position of responsibility for Clinical practices at the SUD treatment center in our community. Our leadership team worked together to establish an improved method for communicating with our local police department and Emergency Room services.

Although none of this was working smoothly and often encountered glitches of one thing or another, everyone involved remained engaged with finding the best possible solution within the circumstances. I think this is one of the benefits of living in a small rural community. We recognize we are all we have and working together makes things easier in the long run. MawMaw often said things like "everything has a value" and reminisced about life during the Great Depression. She said they often bartered fresh eggs or produce from the garden as payment when cash was not available. She was recycling before it became the thing to do.

Michael Meit, senior fellow in NORC's Public Health Research department, Director of Research programs for East Tennessee State University's Center for Rural Health Research and recipient of the 2019 National Rural Health Association's Outstanding Researcher of the Year award is generating recognition for drawing on the strengths of rural communities rather than focusing on deficits and barriers.

Meit, Michael, and Alana Knudson. **"Leveraging Rural Strengths to Overcome Population Health Challenges."** *American Journal of Public Health*, vol. 110, no. 9, pp. 1281-1282.

See also
www.opioidmisusetool.norc.org/
www.ruralcommunitytoolbox.org/

"Rather than focusing so much on rural challenges, I think we really need to tell the positive story about what is good and strong about Rural America."

listen to the full interview www.rhlradio.libsyn. com/170-a-conversation-with-michael-meit

I reached out to him by telephone to inquire about his findings regarding why the highest rates of overdose deaths are within the Appalachian Mountain range communities of West Virginia, Ohio, and at the north end of the Appalachia in New Hampshire. While we were on the phone, he directed me to Google an online tool he created that tracks the rates of overdose deaths (among several other details) by county in every state of the United States. Multiple factors are involved. Reduced employment opportunities where multiple generations have worked such as the coal mines in the southern Appalachians or the paper mills in northern New England. This type of job loss taps into our sense of place and identity.

Find out more about NORC:

We are frequently asked by journalists and others about our name and its proper use in their stories, research reports, and other public situations. Here is the answer to that question:

We were founded and incorporated in 1941 as the **National Opinion Research Center** and this remains our legal name. In 2010, to reflect the many changes in our mission and the global nature of our work, we registered NORC as our externally facing, to-do-business (TDB) name.

We use the name NORC at the University of Chicago for all public, media, and communications purposes. The recommended first reference is "the non-partisan and objective research organization NORC at the University of Chicago," with subsequent references simply NORC. If it is spoken, we say "Norc" as one word.

NORC is not an acronym, it is our name, as with organizations such as IBM, AT&T, RAND, and GEICO. We use NORC at the University of Chicago to emphasize our close affiliation with the University.

Taken on 9/15/20 from www.norc.org/
about/Pages/about-our-name.aspx

One of the things our local Police Department started doing including arriving for emergency transports without running their sirens and lights. When they entered the building their manner was cool, smooth, and approachable. This proved amazingly effective for de-escalating many situations that could have easily become hostile or involve combative behavior.

Other positive changes we have seen since 2016 involve three other very important contributors: a Recovery Friendly Workplace Employer, a free walk-in Recovery Support Center (The North Country Serenity Center), and a long-term sober living community (The White Mountain Recovery Homes).

Untreated addiction costs New Hampshire's economy $2.36 Billion

**66% of that cost ($1.5 Billion) is incurred
by businesses in the form of
impaired productivity and absenteeism - PolEcon Research**

Led by Governor Chris Sununu, New Hampshire's "Recovery Friendly Workplace Initiative" promotes individual wellness for Granite Staters by empowering workplaces to provide support for people recovering from substance use disorder.

The Recovery Friendly Workplace Initiative gives business owners the resources and support they need to foster a supportive environment that encourages the success of their employees in recovery.

Although these three programs are independent of one another, their mission is the same; to serve families in the community by connecting them with recovery support services. The **Recovery Friendly Workplace Initiative (RFWI) is part of the New Hampshire Governor's** comprehensive workforce development plan and specifically targets improving work culture to encourage employees engaging with treatment. Being able to maintain a sustainable workforce is an important piece of the economy.

Mark Bonta talks about his personal experience with nicotine addiction in his interview about the Recovery Friendly Workplace Initiative and starts with a quote *from Dr. Gabor Mate:*

"When I am sharply judgmental of any other person, it's because I sense or see reflected in them some aspect of myself that I don't want to acknowledge".

Addiction is not just about illegal drugs. Smokers, heavy drinkers, and those with behavioral addictions are all in the same boat as hard-core drug users. All of them have the same internal struggle of looking outside of themselves to comfort a pain or emptiness that they developed when they were young.

I started smoking cigarettes when I was twelve years old, and I remain a nicotine addict who struggles in recovery every day. The only difference between me and a hardcore drug user is that the substance I misuse is not illegal. So, who am I to judge? As they say in today's COVID-age, we are all in this together!

> Find Mark Bonta's interview about the
> Recovery Friendly Workplace Initiative in the Turning
> Point Stories & Interview Transcripts.

However, getting a job and keeping a job is just one piece of the reality. For those living with a chronic disease like a substance use disorder, maintaining consistency is tough especially if your living circumstances are not stable or are complicated with other medical issues. This is where the Sober Living Homes offer a practical solution. Working to stay sober and developing new habits for a healthy lifestyle has a higher chance of sustaining long-term change if surrounded by others who share the same goals. We now have enough research validating long-term Sober Living Housing significantly boosts an individual's achievement of sustainable change. This is the foundation for achieving long-term recovery. See the resource list for more information about Sober Living Housing.

> Find the 2020 interview with the founder and owner of
> the White Mountain Recovery Homes in the Turning
> Point Stories & Interview Transcripts.
> More information about Sober Living Homes
> can be found in the Resource section of the Action Guide Workbook.

Proof is in the pudd'n.

RFWI is living proof of how successful management of chronic workplace stressors is possible. The collaboration between RFWI employers and recovery-oriented supports like The White Mountain Recovery Homes and the North Country Serenity Center are positive change agents within our community. These three programs were established as the result of positive legislative action in response to the Substance Use Disorder treatment workforce crisis.

Find the 2020 interview with the Executive Director of the
North Country Serenity Center in the Turning
Point Stories & Interview Transcripts.
More information about Recovery Support Centers
in the Resource section of the Action Guide Workbook.

An Occupational Phenomenon

As mentioned earlier, WHO announced in 2019 burnout is associated with unsuccessfully managed workplace stressors. Burnout is not defined as a medical diagnosis. It is in the category of an Occupational Phenomenon.

In Dr. Sally Garhart's MD interview, she talks about the work culture norm that existed during her early years of development as a physician and while completing the required on-site service delivery. *For twenty years I have acknowledged that I am in lifelong recovery for workaholism and perfectionism and have had burn out in the past. When I began medical school in 1979 at University of Missouri, Columbia there were two hours of academic teaching about alcoholism and addiction during the four years, but the Harry S. Truman Veterans Administration Medical Center where I did a six-week surgery rotation was my lab portion seeing the consequences of decades of drug and alcohol abuse.*

When I rotated through anesthesia as a student and was shivering from the cold, my attending popped an ampule of amyl nitrate into my face Omask which caused me to flush immediately almost falling over. He told me that I had to "feel" how all the drugs worked which absolutely floored me. I remember rounding with a high-risk OB doctor who would drink his patient's three ounce wine cups served with dinner if his patient did not want it frequently, downing twelve ounces in thirty minutes; the patients loved his attention.

On the surgical and some medicine rotations, the attending would take the whole team to a bar after rounds on Friday and buy everyone drinks. It sounds shocking now but those were the norms including Friday night "Liver Rounds" where pizza and beer were served at 5 p.m. in a conference room to students, residents, and attendings lasting until the beer and pizza were gone. I didn't like beer, so I never drank on-call, but others did. There was a lot of post exam binge drinking and drug use in med school. I had female running buddies for my stress outlet.

I saw fellow students and residents take time off, go to treatment, or drop out, but reasons or diagnoses were not discussed. As a third year medical student, I was on call when a fourth-year student whom I knew died by suicide.

The history of labor law and occupational health regulations is beyond the scope of burnout associated with work. However, it does not seem right for me to write a book about worker well-being and not pay respect to my family history and to those who have contributed to moving these issues forward with improvements.

Family History

My grandparents were young adults during the Great Depression. The Great Depression was the worst economic downturn in the history of the industrialized world, lasting from the stock market crash of 1929 to 1939.

My paternal grandfather, "PaPa" George Thomas, worked in the West Virginia coal mines until 1945. My Dad, Franklin D. Thomas, was in eighth grade when they moved to Radford, Virginia where he met my mother, Dolores Bishop. PaPa left working in the coal mines to work for the United Mine Workers of America (UMWA) as an advocate for the improvement of work conditions.

At that time John L. Lewis was the driving force behind the founding of the Congress of Industrial Organizations (CIO), which established the United SteelWorkers of America and helped organize millions of other industrial workers in the 1930s. In 1948, the UMWA won an historic agreement establishing medical and pension benefits for miners. Lewis led the campaign for the first Federal Mine Safety Act in 1952 ("John L. Lewis").

"PawPaw" Norris Bishop is my maternal grandfather. He made his mark on employee welfare in southwestern Virginia as a co-founder of the first Credit Union in Radford, Virginia, where I was born and raised. His career, as with my father's, was in the Steel Industry at the Radford Pipe Shop Foundry. I remember it being referred to as "The Foundry".

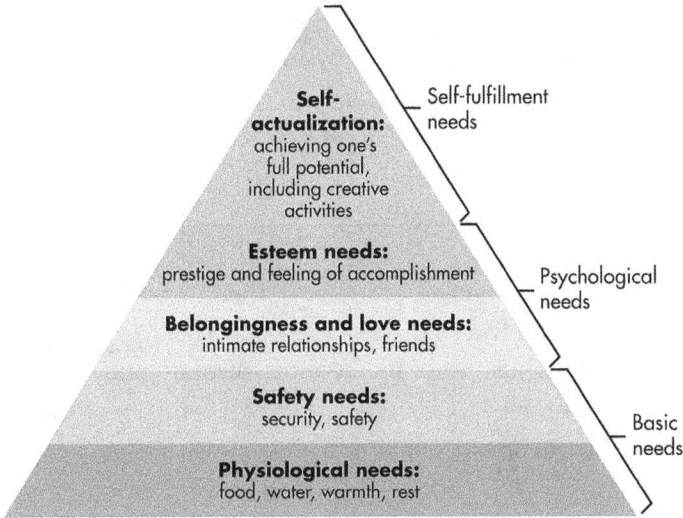

Maslow's Hierarchy of Needs

Safety comes first.

Albert Maslow's Hierarchy of Needs model (1954) is helpful to illustrate the necessity of safety being established first. Here in the United States, standards of practice for workplace safety are considered a norm in today's work culture. The importance of a safe work environment to worker productivity is like the importance of basic need of food, water, and shelter for individual and family productivity. Maslow's Hierarchy of Needs Model is developmental and sequential illustrating each level is dependent on the previous completion for progress to the next level.

    Currently, the global pandemic has pushed our global community into re-defining "what is safe". Now we do not yet have a vaccine, or another means of controlling the COVID-19 progression that is not in conflict with the norms of how the world economy functions. Each of us have unique circumstances defining our level of risk of exposure. At this point one solution that addresses everything is not yet clear.

    Soon after the Pandemic was announced in the United States, **the Larry A. Green Center in Virginia** launched a series of weekly surveys tracking how primary care providers are coping and adjusting. The survey is titled according to the week they are completed, and highlights posted on their website:

"There were 523 clinician participants from 47 states and Guam in Series 17 of our survey, fielded July 24-27, 2020. **Four in five** *surveyed clinicians report practice strain is worse than in March, the first month of the pandemic, with* **50%** *saying that they are just getting used to the poor conditions."*

Necessity is demanding innovation.

As a result of the pandemic, all of us are pushed to find new ways of going about our work and our lives. The survey responses being collected by the folks at Larry A. Green Center could be the most accurate pulse we have now of trends and impact on medical practices. The comments from the above-mentioned Series 17 demonstrate the profound necessity for self-care as an ethical imperative.

Each generation builds upon the achievements established by the previous generation similarly as Maslow's Hierarchy of Needs outlines a developmental process. My grandparent's generation witnessed transition from agriculture economy to industrial.

My PaPa Thomas was motivated by his lived experience working in the West Virginia coal mines to advocate for safer working conditions. My PawPaw Bishop was motivated to improve economic stability for steel workers in southwest Virginia.

PawPaw Bishop was among a small group of steel workers to establish one of the first Credit Unions in southwestern Virginia. This financial establishment is where I opened my first checking and savings account and continue to use Credit Union services.

My father's lifetime career at the Foundry where he held the position of Maintenance Director also responsible for "plant safety". His father, my PaPa, established the first Coalminers Union Office Headquarters in Radford where I was born and raised. The original lettering on his office window can still be seen there on Main Street.

Three things stand out in my memory of PaPa: his deep boisterous and infectious laugh, his large tough hands, and a constant sniffle. Much later, I learned the sniffle is a typical symptom associated with respiratory complications of black lung disease caused by breathing the dust and soot inside the West Virginia coal mines.

Although I do not remember specific events, I do remember lively discussions on the topic of Union activism for worker safety during our visits in their home.

I was a young child when both of my grandfathers died. Although their deaths were separated by several years with PaPa going first, their memorial services were my first experiences with funerals. Besides the awful feeling of seeing them stone cold dead in their caskets during the viewing hours, I remember feeling a sense of awe at the number of people who came to pay their respects. The amount of gratitude these "strangers" expressed has stayed with me my entire life.

This impression was a seed planted in my heart and in my mind that grew to become part of my work ethic belief system. I will say more about this after I finish telling you about my PaPa.

The coal mining industry has a long history in West Virginia. At that time, coal miners did not have access to healthcare benefits or retirement plans. My PaPa did not want his children and grandchildren depending on that history for their livelihood. He died knowing he accomplished that.

I imagine if my Papa were here today and I asked him to comment on the topic of unsuccessfully managed chronic workplace stress leading to burnout, he would laugh out loud, slap his hand on his knee, and say something like, "Dang girl, that ain't the half of it."

His tough hands and that sniffle told the story of his hard-working life. From my child's memory his precious 20% of compassion satisfaction was always there giving him and everyone around him a strong sense of place.

It is fair for me to say advocating for worker well-being is in my blood.

Invitation for Reflection

What or who has influenced your work ethic?

How do your beliefs about work ethic help or hinder your precious 20%?

The Roots of Balance

To keep things balanced, I want to also pay my respects to the women in my family. The Blue Ridge and Appalachian Mountains dominate the Southwestern Virginia landscape. It is one of my favorite places to be during

March mud season in northern New Hampshire. At that time of the year in southern Virginia, the air is full of springtime aromas like fresh cut grass and magnolia blossoms.

My interest in working with plants came from my maternal Grandmother **Josephine Bishop**, my "MawMaw", and my love for quilting and sewing from my Dad's mother **Lily Thomas**, "MaMa".

MawMaw Bishop was a "private duty nurse". At that time, this is what they called nursing care delivered in the private home of someone with a chronic disease in the last stages of their life. This type of nursing care is now part of Hospice Care. Both of my mother's parents grew up in southwestern Virginia in families whose livelihood was defined by the agriculture-based generation. My grandparents grew up during the Great Depression. They lived through the transition of our work culture moving away from the agriculture-based economy and into the industrialized economy.

Work with what you have and make what you have last

My maternal grandparents grew up farming in the Roanoke Valley and Fincastle region of southwestern Virginia. Growing up during the Great Depression made an impression on them about the necessity of how to work with what they had and to make what they had last. Both of their families moved into town where steady and reliable income was available.

Although I never had the pleasure of knowing my mother's grandfather **Parish Hall**, his reputation as a farmer impressed me as a child. While I was growing up, we always had a vegetable garden with green beans and tomatoes. Both my grandmothers mostly cooked from scratch and preserved vegetables and fruits. They always had something prepared on the stove whenever we visited.

Now, every time I put up a jar of applesauce or brew a fresh batch of sweet, iced tea, my grandmothers are with me.

Life Balanced

Not until later in my adult life did I recognize the importance of maintaining this part of my family history. Working with the seasonal cycle of my gardens gives me a sense of groundedness and great pleasure. This is an important part of my daily routine that feeds 20% compassion satisfaction in my work-life balance.

When I first learned about Ayurvedic medicine, my response was dismissive. I recognized many of the concepts as common sense and reminded me of MawMaw Bishop's remedy for nearly everything was a good bowel movement. Many scholars consider Ayurvedic medicine to be the oldest healing science. In Sanskrit, Ayurveda means "The Science of Life" and is often called the "Mother of All Healing."

My twenty-two-year-old daughter has been abroad the past several years and was home recently. She is studying the craft of growing, harvesting, and preparing medicinal plants. Her presence and curiosity about the variety of plants growing at our home reconnected me with the healing capacity of working with plants.

The pleasure of learning from my children is some of the best medicine I can imagine.

Our yard is part of a former dairy farm. We have lots of dandelions, burdock, and mullein, among many other naturalized varieties of plants. During the time of her visit, I developed a nagging cough that felt like something lodged in the back of my throat but would not go down or come out. My daughter reminded me of how these three plants are useful for treating congestion among other symptoms and ailments when dried and prepared as a tea. She helped me re-establish a routine of preparing and using medicinal teas. Again, sometimes family, or close dear friends are the best medicine._

MawMaw's wisdom about the importance of bowel movements has stayed with me. Being aware and involved with the living creatures and plant life surrounding our home has a wonderful way of helping me feel like everything is as it needs to be. Relax. I wonder if I would feel this way if I had grown up in an urban or metropolitan environment? See Herbalism in the Resource section of the Action Guide Workbook.

Burnout crept up on me. I lost touch with my precious 20% during 2016 and 2017. My daily routine of preparing tea and eating breakfast, tending to my gardens, walking in the woods, practicing gentle yoga, playing Frisbee fetch with Panda. I sacrificed all these things and rationalized it as a prioritization of time to focus on financial responsibilities.

I lost my connection to the joy of my work at home and in my job. What is worse, I believed it was necessary. This thinking nearly stole my life right from under my nose.

Invitation for Reflection and Action

Think of a time when you felt worry free and all was well or balanced.

Adjust your posture to an upright vertical position.

Image holding a strand of pearls from end to end.

As you breathe in, imagine this inhalation creating space between each vertebrae of your spine—use the image of the strand of pearls to help your mind see the spaces between each vertebra with each inhale.

As you breathe in, notice how your spine and rib cage work together welcoming the expansion of your lungs as you take in new air.

As you exhale out, notice how your spine and rib cage relax and let go of this expansion.

~ Pause and let this soak in for a moment ~

Is there something you can let go of now to welcome more space into your emotional or physical self?

If you can, identify the first step for allowing yourself to let go of it.

If you cannot, let this go without judgement and invite yourself to remain open to revisit this at another time.

If you like, mark a day and time on your calendar when you will complete this first step.

Hindsight is 20/20 in 2020

Looking back, I can see how I justified letting go of what I considered at the time as non-essential. For example, one of the first things I gave up was my time working outside. The entire act of being outside, engaging with whatever the weather is doing now, walking, hiking, skiing or being quiet to watch the honeybees and birds—all of this is essential. However, at that time, I did not see this and believed I was being responsible, reliable, committed, and loyal.

The Professional Quality of Life measure (ProQOL) was introduced in chapter one. It measures three states of well-being: Compassion Satisfaction,

Compassion Fatigue, Burnout and Secondary Trauma also called Vicarious Trauma. One of the opening statements in the slide presentation available on the ProQOL website explains fatigue is inevitable, therefore it is an ethical imperative to actively engage preventive measures.

Empathy is the ability to be present and without judgement.

Although "bedside manner" is used when describing friendliness and approachability for medical hospital staff, the concept of approachability also applies to behavioral health treatment providers.

Empathy defines our effectiveness as providers of care. Brené Brown, PhD, LMSW is a research professor at the University of Houston Graduate College of Social Work and one of my favorite resources. I rely on her material when I want to share with a client easy to understand material on difficult topics, like changing habits and faulty thinking. Her YouTube clip on empathy is a must-see.

Bedside manner is our ability to be empathetic. Connecting with another person in a meaningful and helpful way is a profound experience. The words spoken are not as important as non-judgmental presence. Brené Brown calls this presence empathy. However, this strength can also be the very source of our burnout if we do not have the ability to protect ourselves from the draining capacity of being a helper.

We Bring Ourselves to Work. Dr. Stamm talks about the concept of bringing ourselves to work to explain how our habits, beliefs, and ways of thinking influence how we interact in the world. Work ethic plays a big role in our work-life balance.

Loyalty, dedication, commitment, reliability, these are some of the words I have associated with defining my work ethic. Dedicated workers do what needs to be done, right? Loyal workers do what is asked of them, right? Reliable workers never back down from a challenge, right?

Dr. Stamm and her colleagues' research show there is a breaking point in the work-life balance. **Any imbalance not addressed and resolved will eventually show up in our work performance.**

Everything in moderation. Work ethic standards that served me well throughout my life became lead weights during the final months leading up to my personal crisis in 2017. The bindings for those weights were expectations of myself that grew into irrational thinking. Irrational thinking produces irrational decisions.

My motivation had become fear driven and based on what I could not control or change. Knowing the difference between what we can and cannot control is the foundation for living in recovery just as safety is the foundation for human development. I lost touch with that foundation.

A groundbreaking study that continues to motivate research to understand how burnout happens, its impact on our healthcare system, and how to fix it was published in 1999 by the National Institute of Medicine, "To Err is Human". As explained earlier, this report revealed evidence that many United States hospital deaths were related to medical error.

The third leading cause of death in the United States is medical mistakes and includes as many as 440,000 preventable deaths every year.

The number one cause of death in the United States is heart disease at 633,842, and cancer is in second place at 596,930.

To understand the complexity of this report and the reality of its impact can be achieved by watching the 2019 released documentary *To Err is Human*. The following statement was taken from the film's introduction: *It focuses on the belief, held by a select few, that acknowledging the current systems' imperfections can lead to its improvement.* Creating systemic improvements ushers in a *new culture of safety in medicine.*

To Err is Human, an in-depth documentary about the silent epidemic of medical mistakes and those working quietly behind the scenes to fix it. Tall Take Productions

---

Producer and Creative Director Mike Eisenberg says this, "We created this film to showcase solutions that are easy to implement and would dramatically improve the quality of healthcare immediately."

The film is dedicated to his father, Dr. John M. Eisenberg, the director of the Agency for Health Care Research and Quality, until his passing in 2002. Dr. Eisenberg is one of the early leaders of patient safety efforts in the United States.

As mentioned earlier, WHO's definition of burnout
begs the question of responsibility

Who or what is responsible for successfully managing workplace stressors?

In 2016, the U.S. Surgeon General's report named Addiction as a National Epidemic. What this meant to myself and my colleagues here in New Hampshire, as mentioned in the introduction, is we are not alone in the North Country. The crisis we had been dealing with was named a National Epidemic. Naming it as a National occurrence validated our experience was no longer something unique to our region of the state. Since then, New Hampshire was and still is third in the nation with the highest number of deaths due to Opioid overdose.

By the time you read this, data will have changed, ie; on July 6, 2020 the POLITICO Magazine published an article titled "US government officials are seeing a rise in methamphetamine and opioid overdose deaths since Global Pandemic was announced".

If you have worked in a situation, regardless of personal or professional, and you constantly don't have enough of whatever you need to do whatever needs to be done, then you know what it's like to be in the company of burnout. Compromises are made to do the best you can with what you have. These problems push us to find solutions or push us somewhere else. This is when that precious 20% earns its weight in gold; the gold being resilience.

Moral Injury

When lives of others are inserted into the equation of need exceeding resources, ethical dilemmas become more complicated. Since contemplating the writing of this book, I have listened to many conversations on this topic and the one that has moved me the most is about Moral Injury (Jameton).

This term Moral Injury was originally associated with combat war veterans experience (Barnes). The word moral is fitting because of the internal conflict between what one believes as "right" and the external demand of following commands, orders, or other administrative requirements.

Most recently Moral Injury is being applied to the healthcare system (Talbot).

I have been honored with opportunities throughout my career to sit in the presence of some veterans and public servants to witness their descriptions of their experiences. The basic training for being a soldier or public safety officer is preparation for killing other human beings. The expectation is to serve, protect, and follow command. Not all situations are equal. Some involve innocent lives being used as a human shield or first responders providing care and assistance to the same location for multiple overdose incidents. These are only a few examples.

> In the 1990's Psychiatrist Johnathon Shay identified
>
> **Three components of Moral Injury.**
>
> (a) There has been a betrayal of what is morally correct.
> (b) By someone who holds legitimate authority; and
> (c) in a high-stakes situation.
>
> Factor (b) is an instance of what Shay describes
> as "leadership malpractice" (Shay).

I cannot help but see this definition of **leadership malpractice** applies to what many are experiencing in the impact of Global Pandemic. For example, during December 2019, the Chinese ophthalmologist, Li Wenliang, who worked at Wuhan Central Hospital issued emergency warnings to local hospitals about mysterious pneumonia cases discovered in the city in the previous week. He was reprimanded by his government authorities. Dr. Wenliang died February 7, 2020 in Wuhan Central Hospital due to what the world now knows as COVID-19 (Davidson).

Addiction Professionals may find themselves at a crossroads when the demands of an organization where the Provider is affiliated poses a conflict with the NAADAC Code of Ethics. Providers shall determine the nature of the conflict and shall discuss the conflict with their supervisor or other relevant person at the organization in question, expressing their commitment to the NAADAC Code of Ethics. Providers shall attempt to work through the appropriate channels to address the concern (NAADAC).

COVID-19 has brought a raft of intense new stressors while removing many of the resources people have traditionally used to cope with stress. But it will be a while before COVID-19's actual impact on the nation's suicide rate is known, says psychologist Jill Harkavy-Friedman, PhD, vice president of research at the American Foundation for Suicide Prevention. "We're two years away from having data," she says. And it is not a given that the pandemic will cause suicide rates to increase, emphasizes Harkavy-Friedman, who is also an associate professor of clinical psychology, in psychiatry, at Columbia University.

"One event can bring stress, but it's not going to make someone suicidal out of the blue," she says, explaining that it is typically a combination of biological, psychological, environmental and other factors that renders people vulnerable to suicide. Take the Great Recession of 2008, she points out. "About 4.8 million people lost their jobs, and the suicide rate didn't skyrocket," she says. "We're much more resilient than we give people credit for" (Clay).

One of the first scholarly publications on the topic of how stress influences well-being was written in 1978 by Charles Figley; *Stress Disorders among Vietnam Veterans: Theory, Research, and Treatment*. Figley is co-founder of **The Green Cross Academy of Traumatology**, the first international organization dedicated to not only helping those impacted by disaster and tragedy but also to the wellbeing of those who serve as first responders. It is an international, non-profit, humanitarian assistance organization of trained traumatologists and compassion-fatigue service providers. Most are licensed mental health professionals; all are oriented to helping people in crisis following traumatic events.

**"If you give a man fish, you feed him for a day.
But if you teach a man to fish, you feed him for a lifetime."**

This was the message from State Senator Laura Boyd, PhD,
and others in Oklahoma City immediately after the first
modern act of domestic terrorism: the bombing of the Murrah
Federal Building on April 19, 1995 (Green Cross).

When mental health professionals like Dr. Boyd were asked what was needed in response to this tragedy, everyone replied "lessons for trauma recovery." They wanted training and competence to assess and treat fellow Oklahomans. Out of this request for help emerged the Green Cross Foundation and the Green Cross Projects.

In September 1997, under the aegis of the Foundation, the Academy of Traumatology was established by Dr. Figley and other leaders in the field of traumatology, including especially Frank Ochberg, Bessel van der Kolk, and Gorge Everly.

Green Cross established Self-Care as a standard of practice:

As with standards of practice in any field, the practitioner is required to abide by standards of self-care. These guidelines are utilized by all members of the Green Cross Academy of Traumatology. The purpose of the Guidelines is twofold: First, do not harm to yourself in the line of duty when helping/treating others. Second, attend to your physical, social, emotional, and spiritual needs as a way of ensuring high quality services to those who look to you for support as a human being ("Standards of Care").

This concludes the first part of this three-part book. This first part establishes the evidence and scientific explanation justifying the importance of self-care as an ethical imperative to quality patient care and safety. Out of curiosity, I researched the symbol of the Green Cross. It is a symbol of nature and life. Green is the best suitable color to represent life in a spiritual sense. Generally, today, a green cross has a secular meaning, and the most common use is health care. In particular, the green cross represents First Aid. I find this to be a delightfully simple and direct way to represent the mission of the GreenCross organization which is to promote and demonstrate the ethical imperative of self-care as healthcare workers. The story of their establishment beginning as the result of tragedy from the terrorist's attack on the government buildings in Oklahoma is yet another example of communities creating solutions in response to crisis.

An ironic side note, in California, the Green Cross name and logo are registered trademarks for the non-profit Public Benefit Corporation, a fully licensed dispensary of medical cannabis in San Francisco.

Contrary to popular belief, the Red Cross is not a public-domain First Aid symbol. The Red Cross of the International Federation of Red Cross and Red

Crescent Societies is an emblem protected under the Geneva Conventions Act and cannot be used without permission. The International Standards Organization recommends that a white cross on green background is used as a First Aid symbol. A variation is a green cross on white field, recommended by ISO, it is still widely recognized as a first aid symbol ("What is Green Cross").

CHAPTER THREE KEY POINTS

Our Work Ethic beliefs are influenced by our family history. Insight into that history and the ability to recognize when our expectations disrupting our work-life balance is necessary in the equation for maintaining the precious 20%.

*****Administrative leadership and workers must work together** to accomplish WHO's definition of "successfully manage chronic workplace stress".

Moral Injury is now being used to describe the impact of ethical dilemmas healthcare workers are facing

*****Recovery Friendly Workplace Initiative** is led by New Hampshire Governor Chris Sununu. It promotes individual wellness for Granite Staters by empowering workplaces to provide support for people recovering from substance use disorder. RFWI gives business owners the resources and support they need to foster a supportive environment that encourages the success of their employees in recovery.

*****Sober Living Homes and Recovery Support Centers** are vital contributors to positive culture change regarding sustainable recovery for individuals, families, and communities.

*Find more details in the Resources found
in the Action Guide Workbook.

PART TWO

Main Solution

Biology of Stress and the Science of Hope

CHAPTER FOUR PREVIEW

The scientific evidence for how we can respond to the biological needs of our body and mind to maintain the precious 20% is reviewed. James Redford's 2016 documentary *Resilience: the Biology of Stress and the Science of Hope* is described as the inspiration for the title of this chapter and the reference for understanding how current medical practices are applying the knowledge gained by the 1997 Adverse Childhood Experiences Study (ACES) to reduce chronic health risks caused by stress and trauma. All this information provides the explanation for how a simple 4-step practice called HomeBase can be a tool for maintaining your precious 20%. Chapter Five presents HomeBase in detail.

Witnessing my colleague's crisis and experiencing my own similar crisis soon after deepened my motivation to dig deeper into what seemed to be a local trend. This chapter focuses on identifying solutions for ourselves as individuals.

The previous chapters outline the problem of burnout, some of the contributing factors, and the question of responsibility in terms of WHO's definition of burnout being an Occupational Phenomenon. As a result of evidence-based research stimulated by the 1999 report *To Err is Human* the healthcare industry has produced additional resources to remedy these challenges including the Quadruple Aim and described in more detail later.

Since the initiation of the Action Collaborative for Clinician Well-Being by the National Academy of Medicine, momentum for positive work culture change is building. Pandemic has accelerated this momentum. The final section entitled Advocacy will address the role of leadership and professional associations.

This section focuses on understanding and harnessing what is biologically uniquely our own and built into our DNA as human beings. The topic of the evolutionary nature of instincts is complex and beyond the scope of this discussion. The following section taken from the 2017 article entitled **The Evolutionary Roots of Instinct** acknowledges that this discussion continues to evolve.

Starting in the 1930s, renowned psychologist B.F. Skinner, then a Harvard graduate student, was influenced by Ivan Pavlov's now-famous notion of operant conditioning. As the founder of the school of psychological theory known as radical behaviorism, Skinner went on to define learning as a product of positive or negative reinforcement. He was sure that all animal behavior arose from learning. By the late 1960s, zoologist Jack Hailman argued that instincts do exist, but they are coupled with some learned elements. Today, a fuzzy dichotomy exists in behavioral science circles, and instinct has become "the fixed and simple component of behavior," says Barron.

Recent research has supported the idea that instinct might be deeply rooted in what are often considered learned behaviors. Another aspect of the serotonin-triggered epigenetic response in young rats to good mothering is changes in chromatin structure leading to higher expression of genes known to be linked to brain cell growth. The resulting increase in neural plasticity may be devoted, at least in part, to enshrining similarly nurturing behaviors in an offspring's behavioral repertoire (Cudmore).

The **biology of stress** and how it is experienced in the body is a mechanism of homeostasis.

Homeostasis is the foundation for defining our innate ability to assume responsibility for our well-being (Lanese).

In the 1870's, Physiologist Claude Bernard described how complex organisms must maintain balance in their internal environment to lead a "free and independent life" in the world beyond. **This concept is introduced as homeostasis** in the book

"The Wisdom of the Body" (Cannon).

Teaching during my Outward-Bound days as a Field Instructor honed my skills for using analogy and metaphors to illustrate what otherwise could easily lose the attention of my audience. I remember my Dad using tools as an analogy for solving problems, you know, something like; *there is a tool for every job and having the right tool can make all the difference in getting the job done right.*

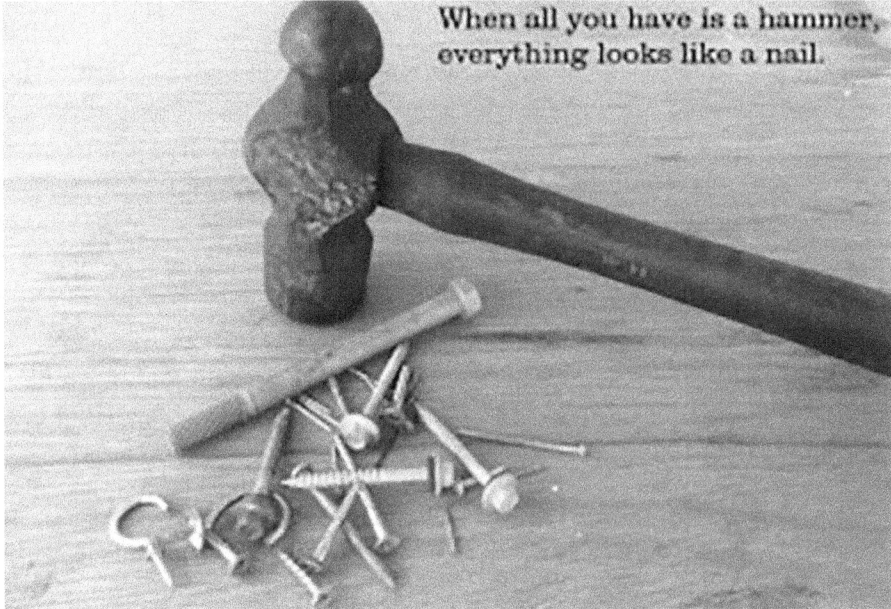

illustration courtesy of sidewaysthoughts.com

Abraham Maslow is credited with being the first to use the phrase

"If the only tool you have is a hammer, then everything is a nail."

The Psychology of Science, 1966, page 15 and his earlier book Abraham H. **Maslow** (1962), Toward a Psychology of Being: "I suppose it is tempting, if the only tool you have is a hammer, to treat everything as if it were a nail".

When teaching clients and facilitating professional development on the topic of affect regulation, I frequently use two analogies relating to prevention and tools.

To understand how to use any tool or instrument or how to repair it, it helps to know how it works. As human beings, our biology is designed to take care of itself. Therefore, it helps if we understand a little bit about how our biology works.

An Ounce of Prevention is Worth a Pound of Cure. Although Benjamin Franklin was addressing fire safety when he used this phrase, it remains true today. Supposedly, during a visit to Boston in 1733, he was impressed with the city's fire prevention methods and tried to bring some of these practices to the city of Philadelphia, where he lived. He sent an anonymous letter to his local newspaper, *The Pennsylvania Gazette.* It was titled "Protection of Towns from Fire" and published on February 4, 1735. The letter began with the expression "an ounce of prevention is worth a pound of cure." Then he outlined an argument for how a city should prepare itself for a fire ("An Ounce of Prevention").

Let us review what we know, as mentioned previously, the Adverse Childhood Experiences Study (ACES) is the largest validated study to date that confirms the link between stress and chronic disease. This study is a robust validation for an ounce of prevention and is worth a pound of cure (Felitti).

Visit the **Center for Disease Control and Prevention** website for downloadable free resources about the ACES, including easy to understand posters illustrating how early childhood experiences impact health, wellness, and mortality.

When teaching, and if I have access to the equipment for playing video clips as well as a reliable connection to the internet, I use a short video clip of ABC Newscaster Dan Harris when he experiences a panic attack while delivering the national news. He has since written two books about what he learned because of that potential career wrecking experience; *Ten Percent Happier* and *Meditation for Fidgety Skeptics* and continues to do some cool things with this material.

I should say, I discovered Dan Harris's material while working for the Department of Corrections running treatment groups. Most of the participants were men. I wanted to find a male voice to represent the mind-body awareness material used in my treatment groups. To this day, I continue to rely on Dan Harris's material to help me communicate complex concepts in a quick and easy to understand format.

Dan Harris: Ten Percent Happier Podcasts
We spend half of our waking lives at work. Get more
focus, clarity, and trust by bringing mindfulness to work.
Brought to you by the world's top mindfulness experts.

Additionally, I want to point out, Mr. Harris also provides testimony to how individual choices can turn our own crisis into an opportunity. The power of a living example is what I know as proof is in the "pudd'n". Most of the people with whom I work, both clients and colleagues, tend to listen to those who have demonstrated through lived experience that they know what they are talking about.

After viewing the entire four and half minute video of Dan Harris's experience, I rewind back to the few seconds we see him panic. His struggle for breath is obvious. His breath pattern looks and sounds like he is sipping short breaths of air.

Everyone can relate to what they see in this short video clip. Seeing Mr. Harris' experience panic immediately engages our empathetic ability to understand. Seeing is believing is taking place in that moment without having to go through a lot of scientific jargon and explanation.

I then review the following images to help explain the mechanics of what Dan Harris was experiencing.

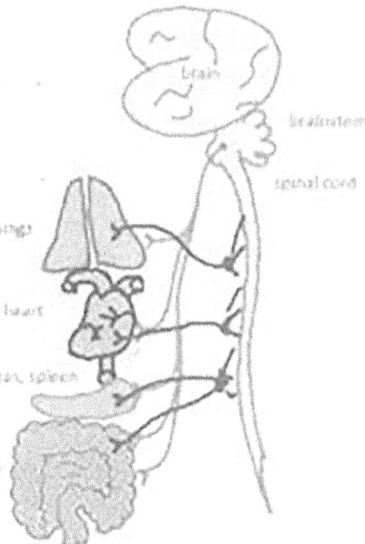

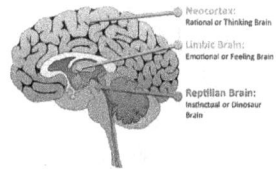

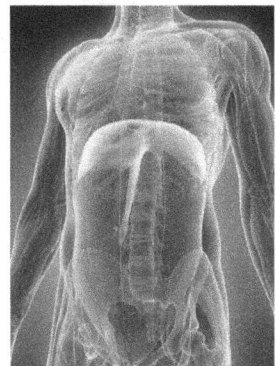

The fight, flight, freeze survival instinct is part of our biological design to prevent the extinction of our species. Through modern technology, science shows us the brain adapts to circumstances as part of that survival instinct; I will explain that concept after first reviewing these diagrams.

First, look at the picture of the torso and notice the rib cage. Inside the image of the rib cage, you can see the diaphragm muscle is drawn up inside of the rib cage. This is an automatic response when the brain perceives a threat. Remember, our biological instinctive drive is to keep the species alive, which means protect vital organs at all costs. The rib cage and diaphragm are the two major protective factors for the lungs and heart.

During Dan's panic, you can see and hear his shortness of breath. This response is caused by the fact his diaphragm is preoccupied with protecting the heart and lungs. If you have ever experienced a full-blown panic attack, you know the feeling of not being able to get a full breath. At its worst, you end up passing out because the brain is not getting enough oxygen to keep you alert.

Reversing the effects of a panic attack on the respiratory and neurological systems you must relax the diaphragm muscle. To do this, inhaling a deep breath is necessary. Think of how many times you have said or heard someone else say, "just take a deep breath…it's going to be okay" However, in the middle of a panic attack it can feel like our brain has stopped thinking, the body has taken over and, in many ways, this is exactly what is happening.

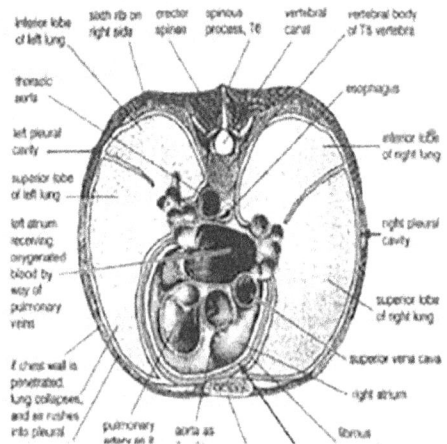

Anatomy of Breathing

D. Coulter, 2001
Anatomy of Hatha Yoga

Our instinctive drive is housed in the lower function of the brain in what neuroscientist Paul D. MacLean identified as the reptilian brain. In his first publication of *The Relaxation Response*, he explains what he calls the Triune Brain. MacLean originally formulated his model in the 1960s and propounded it at length in his 1990 book *The Triune Brain in Evolution*.

The Triune Brain has three major parts: **neocortex** controls our rational and higher functioning or thinking, the **limbic brain** is known as our feeling or emotional brain, and the **reptilian brain** manages our instinctive drives. In times of perceived threat, our instincts take over, prioritizing protection and survival, which results in one of three behaviors, run away, freeze, and try to hide, or duke it out by fighting.

Instincts are not well thought out strategies; therefore, the neurological system shuts down the rational thinking part of the brain. In times of threat, we do not have time to think about what to do. Fortunately, for Dan Harris, his training as newscaster probably included hours of role play and working through various scenarios to prepare him for unexpected events while on the job. The fact he decided to end his report early and transfer the news to his colleagues proves his frontal neocortex was engaged enough for him to make a conscious decision about his behavior rather than succumb to one of the three survival responses.

After his panic attack, the video clip shows him taking several deep breaths and sitting up tall. Again, my guess is his training taught him how to work through moments like that. Fortunately for him, he has leveraged that potentially career wrecking experience into an opportunity to learn and grow from it as he goes on to explain in the remaining portion of that video clip.

The polyvagal theory developed by Steven Porges in 1994, the director of the Brain-Body Center at the University of Illinois in Chicago. Simply put, for the purposes of our discussion, this theory explains the influence diaphragmatic breathing has on the stress response.

Some Stress is Necessary

During the stress response, the brain signals the body to produce stress hormones like adrenaline and cortisol to keep us alert and ready to fight, flight, or freeze. These hormones are a good thing when experienced in moderation. We need a minimal amount of stress to stay awake and remain motivated to complete tasks.

The vagal nerve links vital organs to the spinal cord and contributes to the functioning of the sympathetic and parasympathetic neurological systems. The illustration (insert where to find the illustration) shows the diaphragm muscle attaches to the middle section of the spinal cord.

When the body responds to stress, the diaphragm goes into a protection mode of the vital organs. This protection mode prevents the up and down movement of the diaphragm. This response signals the vagal nerve into the same protection function. To reverse the stress response, the diaphragm must relax and move out of the rib cage down into the belly.

Inhale

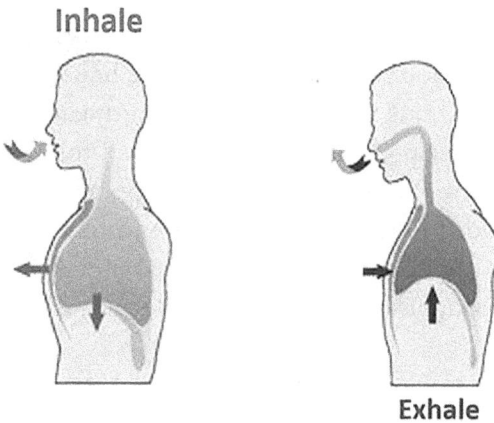

Exhale

If you have ever had the pleasure of watching a healthy baby sleep, you have witnessed diaphragmatic breathing, also called belly breathing, in action. We are born knowing how to do this.

The hard knocks in life teach adaptive behavior.

These coping patterns can end up being maladaptive resulting in problematic behavior such as violence and substance misuse. The movement of the diaphragm muscle up and down the length of the spinal cord acts like acupressure to the vagus nerve. Herbert Benson calls this the Relaxation Response (1976). This relaxation alerts the neurological system into thinking, "Oh, goody, no more threat. We can relax, digest our food, enjoy some music, take a nap, or whatever."

> Step by step instructions for how to elicit the Relaxation Response are found in the Action Guide Workbook.

In the interview with Laura Cooley, she describes her experience with chronic pain and how this led her to discovering her precious 20% solution.

Tell me about your work with the 5-point ear acupuncture protocol & how you became involved. *First and foremost, I suffered with chronic pain for seventeen years despite fifteen years of physical therapists, orthopedists, yoga, Chiropractic care, Rolfing, every kind of bodywork an entry level worker with no health insurance could afford, and I continued to lose ground. With zero help from allopathic medicine, I turned to Chinese Medicine. I do not want anyone to needlessly suffer the way I did, and many people are needlessly suffering. I was partially disabled by the state of Texas. In a state vying for 49th and 50th for least amount of expenditures for human services, that means something. The first acupuncturist I saw gave me Chinese herbs that stopped my continuous spasms. My spasms returned as soon as I ran out of herbs, and I learned about the immense utility and power of Chinese Herbal Medicine. As I had to ride my bicycle fourteen miles to see him, this was unworkable. Why a bike? It was faster than roller skates, my only modes of transportation at the time.*

The traditional medical community provides the primary source of current validated data demonstrating impact of profession-based burnout. Much of this data has been generated by the startling news revealed by the "To Err is Human" report. The National Academy of Medicine's call to action for clinician wellbeing is currently the largest most coordinated effort in the US committed to improving patient care by focusing on providers well-being and is discussed in more detail in the advocacy section.

I am a people person and prefer to work with people rather than numbers. I am not a datastician. However, as a clinician trained to collect history to understand current circumstances and predict risks, I respect and value the importance of knowing the facts. But data does not make sense without understanding its context.

The story I shared earlier about Panda saving my life has enabled me access to delivering important facts and data in a way other people recognize as an authentic effort to make a difference. Citizen efforts to make a difference has proven to be an effective agent of positive change.

For example, the problem of unnecessary deaths due to drunk driver automobile accidents is an example. I often use this example with my clients who come to me as a New Hampshire approved provider of outpatient counseling services required for Driving Under the Influence (DUI) convictions. As a teenager, I can remember the black and red MADD bumper stickers. At that time, drinking alcohol then driving an automobile was considered a norm.

Mothers Against Drunk Driving was a citizen led initiative that gained local and national legislative attention through combining testimony of lived experiences and related facts. Today, the number of deaths due to drunk driving are less.

In my private practice, as a New Hampshire approved provider of the required DUI aftercare counseling, I often share the MADD example to help my clients see the bigger picture of their situation. This explanation for why the regulations and the hoops to jump through exists has worked 100% reducing their complaining about the inconvenience they are experiencing due to their DUI conviction.

In January 2017, the NAM, in collaboration with the Association of American Medical Colleges and the Accreditation Council for Graduate Medical Education, launched The New England Journal of Medicine PERSPECTIVE 313 *To Care is Human: Collectively Confronting the Clinician-Burnout Crisis.* The title causally links it to the original 1999 study that kickstarted two decades of research and investigation to identify solutions ensuring medical error no longer remains the third leading cause of death in the United States.

It was comforting to discover NAM started the National Call to Action for Clinician Well-Being a few months before my 2017 personal crisis. This affirmed that my experience, and that of my two close colleagues the prior year, was part of a larger problem later defined in 2019 by The World Health Organization as an occupational phenomenon.

The World Health Organization (WHO) also announced it will be developing evidence-based guidelines on mental well-being in the workplace. This commitment is based on evidence brought forth since the 1996 World Health Assembly Global strategy for occupational health for all. Currently, an estimated two million people die each year because of occupational accidents and work-related illnesses or injuries. Another 268 million non-fatal workplace accidents result in an average of three lost workdays per casualty, as well as 160 million new cases of work-related illness each year. Additionally, 8% of the global burden of disease from depression is currently attributed to occupational risks ("Healthy Workplaces").

Workers' health, safety and wellbeing are vital concerns to hundreds of millions of working people worldwide. But the issue extends even further beyond individuals and their families. It is of paramount importance to the productivity, competitiveness and sustainability of enterprises, communities, and to national and regional economies.

We must care for what we love.

CHAPTER FOUR SUMMARY

In this chapter the biological function called homeostasis is described as the mechanism for maintaining balance. Better understanding of the three major functions of the brain as described by MacLean's Triune Brain has provided us with better understanding of the fight, flight, or freeze survival instincts. The stress response and relaxation response are defined by Herbert Benson's research. The autonomic functions of our nervous system and their connection with the Vagus nerve explain why diaphragmatic breathing can reverse the stress response. We are born knowing how to breathe using our diaphragm however, these innate abilities can become distorted or replaced by other coping strategies. The good news is we can change unhealthy habits. This research has validated self-care as an ethical standard of practice for healthcare providers. Maintaining self-care practices as part of our professional responsibilities increases our ability to remain in tune with the precious 20%.

CHAPTER FOUR KEY POINTS

The Green Cross Academy of Traumatology was initially organized to serve a need in Oklahoma City following the April 19, 1995 bombing of the Alfred P. Murrah Federal Building. They established a Code of Ethics for Self-Care.

Neuroscientist Paul D. MacLean, MD describes in 1960's **the Triune Brain** with three distinct functions; Reptilian (instinctive drives; fight, flight, freeze), Limbic (emotions), Neocortex (rational thinking)

The Relaxation Response is described in 1975 by Herbert Benson, a Harvard physician, and identifies it as an autonomic reaction that can be stimulated using diaphragmatic breathing and activating the Vagus nerve.

CHAPTER FIVE

HomeBase

> "Emotions are like ocean waves.
>
> They rise and fall every day, every hour, and sometimes, every minute.
>
> Our job in recovery is to learn to surf the waves of our emotions, so we can stay afloat and enjoy life. If we manage our thoughts and feel our feelings, we are able to ride the waves with ease."
>
> Quote contributed by Recovery Warriors
> www.recovery warriors.com/

CHAPTER FIVE PREVIEW

This chapter describes a self-care practice I developed while working for the Department of Corrections. The previous chapter explained the scientific evidence for why and how this simple 4-step practice is effective for maintaining your precious 20%. This practice is called HomeBase and you will read the story of how it got this name. HomeBase can be done anywhere, anytime, and is appropriate to teach your clients, friends, family, and children. The Polyvagal Theory is reviewed and explains the mechanisms of change this simple practice can accomplish.

   Trying to Survive, Focus, and Perform. Two years prior to my spring crisis in 2017, our family experienced several normal expected life transitions. Three of these events involved loss, including the death of my mother. At the time, I was working for the New Hampshire Department of Corrections with responsibility for designing and delivering program material and training and supervising new staff.

On this day, I had recently returned from a second extended family medical leave following the memorial service for my mother in Virginia. Up until then, I had been navigating well; that was my perception.

I was working with an inmate preparing for release. For purposes of respecting this person's privacy, I will refer to them without using personal pronouns like he or she. This was not the first time working with this individual in this setting. I had come to recognize this person to be sincerely interested in positive change and motivated for that change. They had consistently demonstrated good insight and judgement regarding how our individual choices influence our experience. Multiple barriers including finances, employment, housing, and a complex mix of mental health and Substance Use Disorder diagnoses. These realities, even with an affordable comprehensive care plan, are not easily fixed.

My work tasks in that job involved a lot of redundant tasks. Although every situation is unique, the process and steps for moving through the program is designed to be consistent. Routine is important and, in my case, I had become robotic in performing my tasks. I was aware of this and had implemented small little interventions or diversions for myself throughout the day to keep myself entertained and to break up the monotony of my work. I would do things like set up my portable work station in a different location in the room I used, insert selections of music as part of the program for that day, use short video clips to illustrate specific topics for discussion.

One of my favorite video clips to use is called the **Awareness Test** and was originally designed as an advertisement for automobile driver awareness of bicyclists sharing the road. I have noticed there are quite a few spoofs using the same theme. This one is less than two minutes and starts with a group of people dressed in dark and light-colored clothing holding one basketball. The task as viewers of this activity is to count how many times one of the teams passes the basketball while the entire group is moving around.

The scene stops and we are told how many times the ball was passed. Then the narrator says, "But, did you see the moonwalking bear?" The video rewinds and plays again and sure enough, a dude dressed up in a dark furry bear costume moonwalks through the middle of the basketball passing group activity.

**The point is this,
we do not see what we are not looking for.**

Invitation for Reflection and Action

Notice your breath right now as you read this, its rhythm, depth, length of each inhale and exhale

Notice how your body responds to giving your breath attention, i.e.; do you notice any movements in or around your rib cage, belly, under your arms in your armpits, can you feel the sensation of the breath moving in an out of your throat or sinuses, if you are congested pay attention to how your body adjusts to this limitation.

Sit with this for a few moments. Give yourself time to notice what is happening.

When you notice your thoughts evaluating with right or wrong judgements, relax, and let go of the exercise.

Check out what Rick Hanson says about how the mind can change the brain:
www.rickhanson.net/how-the-mind-can-change-the-brain/

What are your thoughts about the mind changing the brain?

On this day, I am feeling particularly distracted and having difficulty staying focused on the tasks at hand.

During my family medical leaves of absence, a lot of sitting was involved. My mother was in late stages of cancer and transitioned onto Hospice Care. If you have experienced anything like this, you know how the pace of activities slows down in these circumstances. To keep myself alert and engaged, I began integrating yoga postures for lengthening my spine, stretching my hips, shoulders, and back while sitting.

To avoid drawing attention to myself, I kept these movements subtle. Up until this day, no one seemed the wiser about what I was doing. But this person caught on and said something to me about it. I remember it clearly because it was like an epiphany for both of us. They said something like this, "Hey, you weren't here and now you are...you did something. I need to learn how to do that. Teach me."

The best way to learn something is to teach it, right?

The previous chapter explains the mechanics involved for understanding why this simple practice can make a noticeably big difference. There are four suggestions or invitations. While you are seated:

Feet flat on the floor
Long Spine
Relaxed Throat
Soft Jaw

6x
Breath 6 rounds of inhale and exhale
exhale 2x as inhale
exhale is twice as long as inhale

Are you doing this yet? If not, give it a try. I will wait.

As mentioned in the previous chapter, Herbert Benson published his research many years ago on the effects of diaphragmatic breathing. His book is called *The Relaxation Response*. Years later, Jon Kabat-Zinn published his findings and called his method Mindfulness Based Stress Reduction (MBSR). Traditional Yogic practice dives deep into using breath control for health and vitality. Today free apps are available to download on your phone for easy access to a variety of ways to enjoy the benefits of breathing. The app called Calm seems to be popular and easy to use.

Jon Kabat-Zinn, creator of Mindfulness Based Stress Reduction said:
"You can't stop the waves, but you can learn to surf."

It is important to remember, to achieve maximum benefit of any exercise, following the protocol for the practice is necessary. In this case, the number six with a lowercase x means six rounds of inhale and exhale and the exhale must be twice as long as the inhale.

> The use of **invitatory language** is important while leading this a group activity or with one person. Use phrases like, when you are ready, when you would like or other phrases that sound like an **invitation rather than a direct order or command.**

David Emerson uses this phrase "invitatory language" in his first book *Overcoming Trauma Through Yoga: Reclaiming Your Body* (2011). The rationale for this is that people living with the negative effects on the ability to trust and feel safe caused by an adverse experience whether it be from a natural disaster, war combat, or a domestic relationship, is the deal breaker on any of this working.

Remember, the mechanism that engages the stress or relaxation response is this autonomic nervous system. We are not in control of this functioning. Our biology is made this way as a survival mechanism. However, our breath is the pathway for engaging change in this system and it works only if we use it. The 12-step slogan *it works if you work it* also applies here.

As discussed earlier when comparing Maslow's Hierarchy of Needs of food and shelter must be met before moving onto higher levels of functioning to the necessity for trust. As leaders, teachers, counselors, parents, and partners, if we do not have the trust of who we are working with, the outcomes of our work will remain shallow.

I should also acknowledge; I have not processed this practice in the traditional academic rigors for qualifying it as an evidence-based practice. Therefore, I use the term evidence informed. This means, what I have learned over the years in my yoga practice teaching and as a student combined with similar evidence-based practices (*The Relaxation Response* and MBSR) have been applied to the HomeBase practice. The effectiveness of HomeBase is a subjective experience.

To clarify further, effectiveness in these circumstances means reduced experience of anxiety, increased ability to focus and concentrate, improved ability to calm oneself when agitated, frustrated, or angry, improved sleep, and an improved general sense of calm throughout the day.

It is simple. We are already breathing. Give it a try.

**"Tension is who you think you should be.
Relaxation is who you are."**

Chinese Proverb

The name HomeBase has a sweet story. The individual who caught me doing this adapted seated yoga practice ended up teaching it to their cellmate. Both attended the groups I offered five days a week. Word travels fast, especially in jail. By the end of that week, the group these two were in, suggested we start and end each group with the breathing practice. After a couple of days of this, one of the people in the group said something like we need to come up with a name for this other than that thing you do in the chair to relax.

After some joking around and batting ideas around, the person who started this, put their hand over their heart and commented about needing to learn how to live "here" while gently patting their heart. The room fell silent. No one cracked a joke or snickered. Then their cellmate spoke up, "Damn dude, you hit that one out of the park...let's call it HomeBase cuz that's what you did...hit it out of the park and can take it easy getting back to HomeBase."

For those of you curious about yoga, the word yoga means to yoke or to bring together the mind and the body. This ancient eastern practice has become popular in the United States and there are many different schools of practice.

The seated posture of HomeBase **is an adaptation** I made from the standing yoga posture called Tadasana. This is the Sanskrit name for Mountain. Sanskrit is believed to be the original language used to record this ancient practice. Many of the posture names are objects found in nature, like Mountain (Carrico). Think about this, 5,000 years ago, the technology of social media, YouTube, television did not exist. People had to work with what they had. In this case, it seems obvious the original yogis were inspired by what they saw around them.

When teaching this, I often use references from our immediate surroundings and the season of the year. For those who are incarcerated, having any time outside, under the sky, and where you can feel the weather on your skin, is considered a privilege. Here in northern New England, all four seasons have distinct differences. In the fall, the foliage can have spectacular color with the Red Maple Trees that grow here. The landscape is remarkable as well. New Hampshire is known as the Granite State for the abundance of boulders and stone here. Granite is used in the foundation and flooring of the jail and I often referred to this as a metaphor to link participants' awareness to the White Mountains of the Appalachian Mountain Range. These mountains are older than those of the west coast and although the east coast has experienced very mild earthquakes, these mountains are more stable and grounded than those resting on earth plate tectonics that are still moving.

HomeBase **goes something like this:**

Imagine yourself standing tall and at ease. Begin your awareness at the bottom of your feet. Notice all your toes, the ball of your feet, the arch, and heal. Your legs and knees are strong and relaxed. Following the image of your spine in your mind's eye, slowly move your attention one vertebrae at a time starting at the base of your spine, your tailbone. While doing this, imagine your spine is like a strand of pearls suspended vertically end to end. As you breathe in, imagine expanding the space between each vertebra to create the sensation of a long and fluid spine. Notice how this is experienced in your body. The intention with this posture is to expand the sensation of your body being tall, strong, and flexible and is not the same as the command to "stand up straight". These words suggest a rigid posture.

What is interesting and delightful, is when practitioners are willing to share their knowledge in the National Association for Detoxification Acupuncture (NADA) collaboration, the benefits are exponential. Most recently, since completing certification training in the NADA 5-point protocol, I have enjoyed collaborating with Laura Cooley and Elizabeth Ropp. We have informally combined simple to do and easy to teach strategies to enable our clients, friends, family, and ourselves to access the natural healing capacity of our mind and body.

Laura has generously shared her expertise with the NADA ear acupuncture protocol at several of the North Country Task Force meetings. Through her innovation and leadership, the Task Force meetings have evolved into a ninety-minute format with at least thirty minutes dedicated to teaching a self-care practice followed by discussion about applications within our unique work settings and work-life balance. Since the original five work groups of the Task Force are now working autonomously, this has been a natural and practical transition for this group, and it remains open to anyone who would like to participate.

Another example of opportunity and innovation being an outcome from the crisis of the pandemic. Elizabeth Ropp speaks in her interview about how the Manchester Community Acupuncture Center adapted to the pandemic social distancing protocols by establishing a YouTube channel. Their website has established a library of short video clips of self-care practices using acupressure. The video clips are four minutes or less and organized by topic.

I suffered from depression as a young adult—things never really came together for me until I moved to New Hampshireand got involved with Community Acupuncturists who are interested in accessibility. I do not tolerate being around assholes very well. I moved to New Hampshire mostly to get away from a bad work situation. It was a great decision. I work on a good team, and I have been able to get involved in local politics.

A seed was planted in 2010 when I interviewed for the job I have now at the Manchester Acupuncture Studio. During my interview with my current employer, Andy Wegman, he mentioned his interest in working on a bill to change legislation to enable more people access to ear acupuncture. That really impressed me.

Diaphragmatic breathing combined with the NADA 5-point protocol has the potential of boosting the benefits of both practices. This breathing practice stimulates the vagus nerve. The vagus nerve is the longest nerve in the body. It originates in the brain as the cranial nerve and travels from the neck and passes around the digestive system, liver, spleen, pancreas, heart, and lungs. This nerve is a major player in the parasympathetic nervous system, which is the "rest and digest" part and functions opposite to the sympathetic nervous system which is "fight or flight".

Check out this resource for evidence-based research demonstrating the effectiveness of the NADA 5-point protocol
acudetox.com/wordpress/wp-content/uploads/2014/07/
Research_Summary_2013-2.pdf

CHAPTER FIVE SUMMARY

Laura explains the efficacy of the 5-point protocol like this: it is more about what it allows to happen than what it does. When I heard her say that I immediately remembered the NYC Fire Chief in her DVD Unimagined Bridges. His department was one of the ground zero responders to the Twin Towers disaster on 9-11. In the interview he talks about his experience with the ear acupuncture and explained he didn't notice any changes for the first day or so and then said he slept well for the first time since the terrorist attack which had been, at that point, several weeks. His comment was, "I don't really care about how it works or why, it works and that's good enough for me." It is simple; if it works, don't fix it.

I originally developed HomeBase for myself. As the story is told, one of the inmates I was working with at the time recognized I had done something to improve my focus and attention. That was the beginning of HomeBase. Teaching something certainly is a great way to know how to do something and that is the outcome of HomeBase. The simple 4-step process was created as a way to help others not otherwise interested in sitting in a chair and breathing for an entire hour. The science currently available with creative video clips make it a fun and easy way to understand how to fine tune the instrument that is our body. HomeBase teaches us how to engage our built-in neurobiological functions to work for our benefit rather than the stress response running us raged. This is yet another way of cultivating our precious 20% compassion satisfaction.

CHAPTER FIVE KEY POINTS

The United States has the highest rate of incarceration in the world (937 per 100,000 adults) (Fox).

A significant and growing number of people in the criminal justice system have co-occurring mental health and substance use disorders. For example, **over 70 percent of offenders have substance use disorders,** and approximately 17–34 percent have serious mental illnesses—rates that greatly exceed those found in the general population

("Substance Abuse").

Highest risk for relapse after release from incarceration is during the first two weeks after release (Ren).

Applying scientifically proven practices can be simple and easy.

HomeBase is an evidence-informed practice that stimulates the vagus nerve. This nerve is important because it is a major player in the parasympathetic nervous system, which is the "rest and digest" part and functions opposite to the sympathetic nervous system which is "fight or flight".

CHAPTER SIX

Start Where you are and Work with What you have

> "Do what you can, where you are, with what you have."
>
> *Teddy Roosevelt*

Quote contributed by Tonya Tavares, MS, CCRP
Assistant Project Director, Brown University School of Public Health, Center for
Alcohol and Addiction Studies, Technology Transfer Specialist for the Opioid
Find Tonya's full interview in the Turning Point Stories & Interview Transcripts.

CHAPTER SIX PREVIEW

My colleague Elaine Davis and I introduce our collaboration as the Healthcare Workgroup, one of the five North Country Task Force Workgroups. Currently, we are several months into the second year of this two-year study. I will briefly review the development and background of this project. You will become acquainted with the New Hampshire Board of Licensing credentials for SUD treatment providers and our role as Board approved Supervisors for the professionals seeking one of these credentials or retaining them. By the end of the chapter you will have a good understanding of the Certified Recovery Support Worker (CRSW) role in addressing SUD treatment needs and the paradigm shift associated with this recent addition to New Hampshire's workforce. Additionally, Elaine introduces herself and describes some of the unique history of SUD treatment in the North Country.

Both of us are approved Clinical Supervisors for the New Hampshire Alcohol and Drug Counselor (LADC) and the Mental Health Practice Licensing Boards. Together we are responsible for the supervision of approximately thirty CRSW candidates as well as providing required supervision for credential retention.

Of the four credentials governed by the New Hampshire LADC Board, the Certified Recovery Support Worker (CRSW) is growing most rapidly. In 2011, four CRSW were on the LADC Board list. In less than ten years, that number has grown to seventy-three making it the fastest growing among the other three groups of professional credentials.

As mentioned previously, the 2018 North Country Provider Needs Assessment identified areas of need in our SUD treatment workforce. Although our numbers are small in the North Country, the message from the data speaks volumes and fueled the momentum of our regional courageous conversations to reach beyond the North Country.

To refresh your memory of the prior mentioned Provider Needs Assessment, the outcomes included ninety-six percent of the respondents met at risk criteria for burnout. Less than forty-five percent of the respondents reported having a supervision agreement and none of them reported talking about their symptoms in supervision because they feared loss of job security.

Additionally, you will recall from the first section in the book, since 2016, **New Hampshire has been only third to Ohio and West Virginia in total number of deaths due to Opioid Overdoses** in the entire United States of America. Despite noble efforts from our Governor and legislative action, our workforce growth has not been able to keep up with the demand for SUD treatment. The Provider Needs Assessment outcomes reflect the drugs continue to win.

Earlier this year, 2020, Wendy Welch, the Executive Director of the Graduate Medical Education Consortium of Southwest Virginia edited and published a collection of stories from doctors, nurses, and therapists dealing daily with the opioid crisis in the southern Appalachia region. This is the region where I grew up as a child and where most of my family remains.

From the Front Lines of the Appalachian Addiction Crisis is yet another affirmation that our North Country regional outcomes from the Provider Needs Assessment are not isolated experiences.

**From the Front Lines of the Appalachian
Addiction Crisis: Healthcare Providers
Discuss Opioids, Meth, and Recovery** (2020)

Stories from doctors, nurses, and therapists dealing daily with the opioid crisis in Appalachia should be heartbreaking. Yet those told here also inspire with practical advice on how to assist those in addiction, from grassroots to a policy level. Readers looking for ways to combat the crisis will find suggestions alongside laughter, tears, and sometimes rage. Each author brings the passion of their profession and the personal losses they have experienced from addiction, and posits solutions and harm reduction with positivity, grace, and even humor. Authors representing seven states from the northern Coalfields and southern Appalachia relate personal encounters with patients or providers who changed them forever. This is a history document, showing how we got here; an evidenced indictment of current policies failing those who need them most; an affirmation that Appalachia solves its own problems; and a collection of suggestions for best practice moving forward.

Editor Wendy Welch is the Executive Director of the Graduate Medical Education Consortium of Southwest Virginia where she advocates for social justice and policy planning in equal measure.
She lives in Wytheville, Virginia.

As Supervisors, Elaine and I have been concerned about the risks of harm for everyone in this equation of SUD treatment workforce shortage. Our lived experience as people in long-term SUD recovery has been, for several years, a strong gut feeling. This dual role of knowledge gained from lived experience and knowledge gained from professional training can be a double-edged challenge.

Both of us got our start in recovery through the Traditions of the 12-Step Self-Help program of Alcoholics Anonymous. One of the Traditions talks about not making any decisions, changes, or starting new relationships during the first year of recovery. Compromises are often necessary when dealing with a crisis. Due to the New Hampshire SUD workforce shortage, compromises have been made to meet the demand for treatment.

One of the compromises both of us have witnessed and involved in trying to mitigate has been hiring SUD treatment staff with less than one-year of sobriety. Over time, we have seen this become problematic for the individual as well as for the employer resulting in a variety of challenges and consistently feeding rapid turnover of staff.

This combined with my own crisis and that of our close colleagues became motivation to invest ourselves in what we believe could be a piece of the solution for this complex issue.

Prior to my involvement with the NHADACA Board of Directors as the Ethics Committee Chairperson, Elaine held this position. The Committee had been inactive for several years by the time I became involved. Her insight and history on this Committee was of great assistance to me in taking on that responsibility. Chapter nine will address these details.

Peer Recovery Support services represent a paradigm shift in the treatment of SUD. William White, the author of *Slaying the Dragon: The History of Addiction Treatment and Recovery in America*, and Senior Research Consultant at Chestnut Health Systems and Associate Director of the Behavioral Health Recovery Management project discusses this paradigm shift.

White says using the term 'peer' rather than 'consumer' encourages this shift. The latter implies support services provided by someone who is or has been a recipient of professionally directed treatment services. In the addiction's arena, recovery support services may be provided by persons in recovery, or otherwise defined as an ally by those receiving help, who have not been "consumers" of treatment services.

Use of the term 'peer' rather than 'consumer' reinforces there are multiple pathways to recovery, not all of which involve professionally-directed addiction treatment, and affirms an identity linked to a community of recovering people rather than a treatment institution. These groups are referred to as 'mutual-aid' groups rather than 'self-help' groups as they technically are not self-help, but an admission that efforts at self-help are exhausted, requiring a reliance on resources and relationships that transcend the self (White).

As Clinical Supervisors of the fastest growing field of practice in SUD treatment, it was a no-brainer for us to figure out how to help address the challenges the New Hampshire SUD treatment workforce is facing.

The data from the North Country Provider Needs Assessment provided us the proof of what our gut had been telling us.

As mentioned earlier, less than 45% of the respondents of the North Country Provider Needs Assessment reported receiving supervision and they are not talking about their burnout symptoms with their supervisor. Fear of losing their job was identified as the primary reason. This is not acceptable. **The good news is this is something we can change.**

Validated evidence-based research has established the work performance of worn out, fatigued, burned out workers increases incidents of harm to patient care and safety. The solution seems obvious. However, recognizing the need for change and engaging what is necessary to make the change is easier said than done, right? For example, global pandemic has everyone frantic for a quick fix. Until a vaccine or some other proven method for preventing the spread and progression of the COVID-19 is established, we have no clear answers for how to protect our kids if they go back to school or protect ourselves when we go back to our jobs. Economic needs conflict with health and well-being, an ethical dilemma with no easy answer or quick fix.

Supervision and Peer Collaboration are mechanisms for risk management in SUD and mental health treatment practices. This process is built in the regulations and the codes of ethical practices. The National Association for Alcohol and Drug Abuse Counselors (NAADAC) also includes expectation of supervisors utilizing the most current resources available is also clearly stated in addition to the prior mentioned self-care practices.

One of the calls of duty in the Substance Use Disorder treatment providers Code of Ethics regarding the role of Supervision and the Supervisor is to engage the most recent evidence-based standards of practice. Elaine and I believe instruction and techniques for Supervision are no longer adequate at managing the risks and challenges we are facing in this Epidemic and now Pandemic. We have committed ourselves to discovering a better and more effective approach to the Supervision process and especially tailored to the CRSW role in the SUD treatment continuum.

> **National Alcohol and Drug Abuse Counselors Association Code of Ethics** (NAADAC, 2016)
>
> **Principle VII: Supervision and Consultation - 24 Current**
>
> Educators and site supervisors shall ensure that program content and instruction are based on the *most current knowledge and information available* in the profession. Educators and site supervisors shall promote the use of modalities and techniques that have an empirical or scientific foundation.

In New Hampshire, the primary difference between Peer Collaboration and Supervision is liability. Peer Collaboration is exactly what it sounds like, professional colleagues meeting together for the purpose of discussing their work. It is a confidential setting where collaborating on ideas for treatment and sharing insight with the purpose of helping one another provide the best possible quality of care to our clients.

Supervision involves a power differential between the one providing the supervision service and the one receiving it. Ideally, a formal Supervision Agreement is established at the onset of the relationship clearly defining responsibilities of both parties. In New Hampshire, this is a requirement for those working toward licensure. The Supervisor assumes legal responsibility for the practices performed by the supervisee. This regulation is in place to protect the public from harm.

Many years ago, I learned about leniency bias, also called leniency error. I was attending a Supervision training led by Dr. Janine M. Bernard who established the Discrimination Model (1979) of supervision and has published more than fifty books, book chapters, and professional journal articles in clinical supervision. After hearing the description of leniency bias, I completely understood. I remember chuckling and thinking to myself, "Oh, yeah, right, we do this all the time. Let each other off the hook for one reason or the other," all of which is beyond our present topic.

I mention leniency bias because it is an accurate title for the behavior it is describing. When confronting anyone with an accountability issue, I can't recall it ever being easy regardless of it being who left the lid off the peanut butter in our kitchen at home or making sure clinical records accurately reflect billing records at work. In the process of delivering supervision services,

I have found referring to leniency bias when addressing accountability concerns with my supervisees has been helpful at reducing the sting of criticism.

Leniency error

is a type of rating mistake in which the ratings are consistently overly positive, particularly regarding the performance or ability of the participants. It is caused by the rater's tendency to be too positive or tolerant of shortcomings and to give undeservedly high evaluations. Also called leniency bias ("APA Dictionary").

Elaine and I are in the second year of a two-year study testing supervision practice tools to address provider fatigue and burnout. We hope the outcomes and lessons learned will contribute to developing a resilient and sustainable SUD treatment workforce here in New Hampshire. The goals of this project are to identify supervision practice effective at appropriately identifying worker fatigue, and provide effective response and management of challenges that come with fatigue.

Thus far, one of the challenges we recognize and continue to encounter is leniency bias. It is our observation much of this bias is rooted in work culture norms unique to peer-based services. Although we have not collected all the data at this point, we recognize addressing this bias upfront at the start in the Supervision Agreement is proving to be a positive change agent in this dynamic.

The first time I heard about leniency bias, I was attending a multi-day Supervision training lead by Janine Bernard, PhD, the developer of the Discrimination Model of Supervision (1972). She prefaced her explanation by identifying the assumption most of the people in the helping profession are "care-takers" who tend to put the needs of others first. Quite a bit of research has gone into this and is beyond the scope of this book. However, I mention it because I recognize this dynamic as well.

Teeter and Ludgate refer to this in their Practical Resilience Workbook (2014) as a potential risk for compromising self-care. Elizabeth Stamm, PhD, the developer of the Professional Quality of Life measure, also refers to this type of risk as "we bring ourselves to work". In other words, people in the helping profession tend to give one another slack when it comes to accountability. Unfortunately, when this is left unchecked, the outcomes lead to unintended compromises to quality of care and potential violation of our first call to duty, do no harm.

Early on in this Supervision project, Elaine and I recognized we needed help with the management of the data we are collecting to protect its validity. After many months of researching potential sources of technical assistance, we established a partnership with Gloo, "a network of individuals and organizations in Boulder, Colorado obsessed with revolutionizing personal growth." When we asked Steven Millette, the Executive Director of Gloo, to explain the meaning of this acronym, he sort of laughed and explained it is not an acronym but rather a play on words representing pulling together and keeping together all the parts that enable programs to be effective and sustainable.

The phrase *obsessed with revolutionizing personal growth* on the Gloo website grabbed our attention. We are hopeful, with their expertise we will be able to provide validated evidence for contributing to updating Supervision practices to carry our SUD treatment workforce development into a sustainable and resilient future.

> *And together, we are building the world's first*
> *personal growth platform built to serve Champions—*
> *the helpers, leaders, and motivators*
> *who work tirelessly to strengthen their people.* www.gloo.us/about-us

Now, I want to introduce you to Elaine Davis. She will wrap up this chapter with a brief review of her history and four decades of providing SUD treatment in the North Country of New Hampshire. Both of us are approved Clinical Supervisors for the New Hampshire Alcohol and Drug Counselor (LADC) and the Mental Health Practice Licensing Boards. Together we are responsible for the supervision of approximately thirty-five CRSW candidates as well as providing required supervision for credential retention.

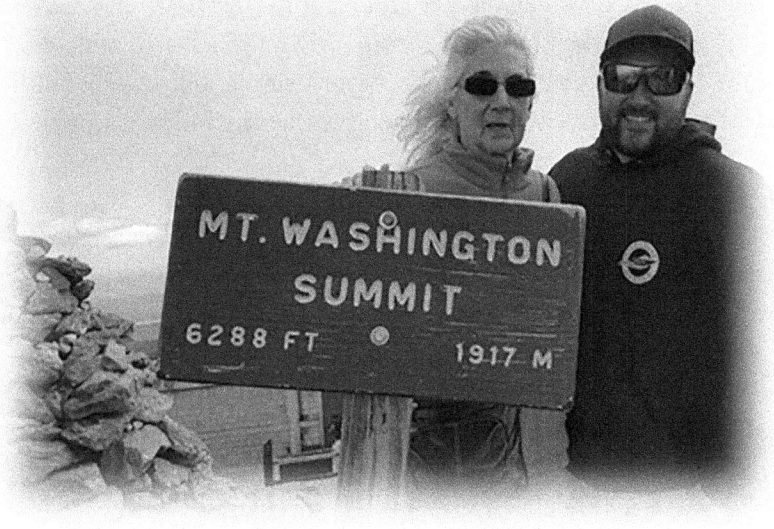

Elaine Davis of Shelburne, NH
Photo taken July 2019 on Mt. Washington summit
with Tyler Brisson, her grandson

Elaine is among the founding members of the North Country Task Force and one of the most consistent voices in these courageous conversations. She was one of the first people to introduce herself to me after I moved north from Dublin, New Hampshire to Bethlehem. She was involved in nearly everything I was interested in knowing more about. She is one of the first colleagues I reached out to as part of my recovery plan after my near suicide attempt.

> Go to the Turning Point Stories & Interview
> Transcriptsto find Elaine's full story.

She also has a long and productive track record serving on the Board of Directors for the New Hampshire Association for Addiction Professionals (NHADACA) and has received numerous awards in New Hampshire for her dedication to serving her fellow human beings.

When introducing ourselves in groups or as part of our presentations, I often say I have been following her around for thirty years and consider her one of my mentors. Her response consistently reflects her humble demeanor and mutual respect as a colleague. We share a similar quirky sense of humor, practice a holistic lifestyle, consider ourselves fiercely independent, and identify the North Country as our home.

Prior to COVID-19, we frequently carpooled to the southern part of the state for training, conferences, meetings, whatever. She lives about an hour north of me and I live about two hours north of where most of these things take place. Now, instead of carpooling, we "Zoom", text, email, and use the telephone—a lot.

August 15, 2020 Interview with Elaine Davis, LCMHC, MLADC

Why did you become a SUD treatment provider? Please share how this happened. *I moved from Plymouth, Massachusetts in 1980 with my two children, then ages six and nine. I had remarried after divorcing my first husband 3 years earlier. I had visited the White Mountains of New Hampshireand believed that it would be a nice place to raise children and get away from the hustle/bustle of Southeastern Massachusetts. It was not exceptionally long before I experienced what I call "cultural shock in reverse" as everyone was Caucasian. I honestly did not see a person of color for over a year. I was involved in A.A. at the time with three years of recovery from SUDs. I was employed as a housekeeper for the well-to-do in the local area. The stark contrast of the busy town I moved from and the crowds of people was very apparent. In general, folks had more of a laid-back attitude, strong work ethic, and more of a respect for nature and the land. I did grow up in a very rural community in Massachusetts, but my experience as an adult was quite different.*

Fast-forward to 1985. My second marriage was in chaos and, by 1986 I was divorced for the second time. My daughter had moved back to her father's in Massachusetts at age ten but returned to live with me in eleventh grade. My son had also moved back to his father's, age twelve, but stayed living in Massachusetts with regular visits. My daughter and I rented an apartment together. My recovery had progressed to allow me to remove myself from another toxic relationship. It was during this time frame that I had a true Spiritual Experience because of a transcendental meditation I engaged in. It did take me many months to unwrap the impact, which stayed with me for three days. Ultimately, I perceived that it meant I was on the right path and that I had nothing to worry about. It is difficult to put into human words the outcome of a Spiritual Experience! Shortly after this experience, I received a call from the Clinical Director of Derby's Lodge Treatment Facility in Berlin, New Hampshire, asking if I would be interested in coming to train as a counselor with them. I was excited and scared at the same time! And so, my career began in 1986. I went back to school the following year, completed my Bachelor of Science degree and my initial Master of Science degree in 1991.

I would like to give a brief history of Derby's Lodge. *Initially, Derby's Lodge was a hunting camp along the Androscoggin River in Dummer, New Hampshire. It was purchased by Tri-County Community Action Council's Director (TCCAPC), Larry Kelley, as he had an incredibly soft heart towards assisting individuals wanting recovery from SUDs. The original Derby's Lodge was staffed, held mutual aid support groups, and housed eight men. Within a short timeframe, the opportunity came up in Berlin, New Hampshire to purchase a three-story building. Tri-County CAP purchased the building and moved Derby's Lodge Residential Treatment to Berlin, New Hampshire. This happened about eighteen months before I began working there. The building housed the Impaired Driving Program, Outpatient Counseling, and residential treatment for thirteen males and six females. In 1991 (possibly 1992), TCCAP purchased the Friendship House Retreat Center in Bethlehem, New Hampshire for the expansion of Derby's Lodge. There was over a year of remodeling to accommodate the program and they kept all staff employed providing some of the assistance to the construction and remodeling. There was also a decision made to adopt Friendship House as a new name for the treatment facility and the name of Derby's Lodge was dropped. The ancillary programs of the company, other than the residential program, remained in Berlin, along with opening a Social Detox for potential applicants who might apply to Friendship House to have a safe and supportive atmosphere while on a wait list. There were many who went to this program because they were homeless, in legal trouble, and/or looking for treatment. The Androscoggin Valley Hospital was in the same town, which allowed for the Social Detox to access immediate medical care should it be needed for any of the residents. They did hire a Medical Doctor earlier before the move who came in and taught a rotating Medical Aspects of Addiction to the residents. She remained the Medical Doctor, along with the move to Bethlehem for the residential program, for over twenty years. I believe this brief history is not only important due to lack of services above the Notches, but to solidify the earlier movement of like-minded individuals who had this vision and were able to financially support the vision.*

My career as a clinician has taken me in many different vocational directions over the years. *More than half my career has been in Private Practice in the Berlin and Gorham areas of New Hampshire. Over the years, I worked for several different companies but usually returned to my private practice. I believe I achieved lasting change in some of the organizations as an employee in different roles. While at a medical facility, I developed, coordinated, and facilitated a pre-natal substance abuse screening and early intervention program. I was also hired as the initial therapist for Founders Hall Outpatient - New Hampshire. There was no other staff hired for almost a year, so I took on all duties. Founders Hall was a part of Northeastern Regional Hospital in St. Johnsbury, Vermont. They had inpatient treatment as part of the hospital, and it was their Director who literally found me through his resources and hired me. Ironically, it was a week after I resigned from a previous position and had no idea where I would work. This was in the mid-1990s. I was employed there until 1993 when I began my private practice. In the late 1990s, I worked for a local hospital as Director of Social Services. Although I was only there for about a year, I was able to lead a team that resulted in an updated, integrated hospital-wide discharge planning policy. There were other positions over the years, but none beyond three years. I often was at odds with management decisions, despite proven methods to the contrary. I often felt badly for workers whom, as mid-management, I would have to deliver upper management's plans. My husband and I, for a few years, experienced the impact of the 2008 recession. This hit the North Country in New Hampshire about 2009 and my husband, a self-employed contractor/builder, was not making the money he used to. He was hardly working, as jobs had dried up for a couple of years.*

In 2012, *my husband's back issues resulted in his applying for early SSI and I believed I needed to make a change in my income. It was that week that a colleague called me from Friendship House and asked if I knew of any MLADCs looking for work, as they were hiring a Clinical Director and needed the advanced licensure. So, it was personal income that solidified my acceptance of this position. I began Clinical Supervision prior to the Clinical Director at Friendship House, but this position formalized me as a Supervisor. I was employed at this position for exactly four years. When I began this position, Friendship House was supported through New Hampshire state funds reimbursement. I clearly remember being asked after about 8 months on the job what my thoughts were about the future of Friendship House, as they were always in the red financially. My answer was simple—"You either grow or close down."*

In 2013, I organized, along with the managing administrator, applications for New HampshireMedicaid certification and commercial Health Insurance companies for reimbursement. This process was tedious and, initially, an administrative assistant was savvy enough to take this roll on and did a great job. The complication came when we became certified by Medicaid and a few other Commercial Health Insurance companies. I understood contracting/billing from my years in Private Practice, even though this was a larger entity, the process was the same. So, I embarked on teaching them about the billing process, to include training of staff, and stated clearly to management that I would set this all up, but once running, I should only be involved in the billing about five-to-ten percent of my time. They assured me they were going to hire a biller and that the staff they temporarily put in place to assist me with this process would be able to be relieved of this duty. Ultimately, this never happened, and, in December 2015, I gave a six-month notice, as I knew I was completely burned out due to lack of resources. My largest concern was the impact on staff (who had no choice) and client welfare. My last day at Friendship House was June 30, 2016.

My next position was as an Independent Contractor for New Hampshire Health and Human Services – Department of Child, Youth, and Families (DCYF), providing expertise and FT assistance working with those experiencing a Substance Use Disorder and had entered the DCYF system through Family Court. I was employed for this Independent Contractor position until June 30, 2019. A few months earlier, I had already engaged in accepting a position to supervise Certified Recovery Support Worker (CRSW) candidates for a new grant-funded program that began July 2018. My contribution to the North Country and my many years (on-and-off) as a New HampshireAlcohol and Drug Counselors Association (NHADACA) Board member, have resulted in numerous recognitions. I have awards from the local Domestic Violence organization, New Hampshire Coalition on Substance, Abuse, Mental Health, & Aging, New Hampshire Attorney General/ Office of Victim Assistance, and several others. In 2014, I received a couple of awards from New Hampshire Alcohol and Drug Counselors Association. I must state, the Lifetime Achievement Award really impacted me. I believe my career was driven by my desire to share recovery, staying on top of the Science of Addiction, resisting those who did not believe in changes within the profession, and client welfare. This award brought home to me the reality that I did make a difference in my many years of perseverance.

I had become familiar with the CRSW profession about 2014 while at Friendship House. I was extremely skeptical at the time, as I believed the hiring *and training of those in early recovery to assist others in recovery was a mistake. Today, I realize I was wrong, as I now understand this position as CRSW, which has since been better defined through New Hampshire legislatures and formal, in-depth regulations. At the same time, the gold-standard for treatment, mostly Opioid Use Disorders, had become Medication-Assisted Treatment (MAT). I had been very ambivalent from the introduction of MAT, knowing full well that clients may have to either stay on this medication for their life or need to go through withdrawal to stop MAT. My opinion today is still skeptical. This is mostly because I see the classic healthcare system placing individuals on medication with extraordinarily little treatment for their issues, they will need to address to truly experience recovery. There are a few organizations that mandate counseling, but many say they are getting treatment, when it seems they only check in for fifteen to twenty minutes with a clinician.*

Today, I am self-employed PT (semi-retired) for this grant-funded program, Strength2Succeed *(S2S), which is the only "bricks and mortar" program funded through the grant in NH, although services can be requested throughout the state by DCYF and other individuals through Granite Pathways, who will provide a clinician to assist in referral issues. This program is a wonderful achievement in the North Country. The Family Resource Center took this endeavor on, hired good people to manage, who are open-minded and caring. S2S hires applicants based upon the criteria of being in SUD Recovery and having experienced a DCYF case. In many ways, this exemplifies a years-long idea that clients who are at their most vulnerable time in their life, are more open to listening to people who have experienced what they are currently experiencing. I currently supervise about fourteen CRWS in various stages of certification and learning their positions through a lot of workplace Reflective Supervision, team-building, and Clinical Supervision. It is paramount with many positions I've had and is best described as "the toughest job you'll ever love"!*

My last comment relates to the Field of SUD Treatment. *Over the years, there have been a lot of avenues, modalities, and changes that have come along with modern society. I laugh sometimes at how the Addictions field was decades ago, but we all did the best we could based on the knowledge and science at the time. There is so much that needs to change in the treatment industry beyond the current systems. SUD treatment needs to be data driven like any other medical condition. There needs to be a better national effort to reduce the stigma of Mental Health and SUD conditions, eventually being more accepted like other chronic medical conditions. Treatment should be available to everyone, especially to fam-*

ilies in need. SUDs are also a family illness, as the impact falls directly on those closest to those experiencing a SUD and therefore, also need recovery. This is not part of a national discussion and mutual aid groups like A.A. and N.A., who have programs like Alanon for families, do not have the attendance or impact they used to due to the advancement of MAT. The traditional medical industry desperately needs changes at the schooling level that introduces SUD as a medical condition that needs treatment. For years, although it may be changing some, doctors had six hours in medical school related to SUDs. There should be a whole course, at minimum, for all medical practitioners before they specialize. The pharmaceutical industry has begun paying large amounts of money for profiteering and misleading providers and clients. However, there is not enough being done to address this impact on families and communities.

Lastly, but not least, we need to acknowledge the time frame it takes for those impacted by a SUD. Treatment needs to be revamped. **When I started my recovery in 1977, it was a different world.** *In many ways, it has only expanded what was already there. Along with incorporating science, Ryan Hampton in his book "American Fix" (2018) has a nice blueprint embedded within the book. He talks about what I have always known that what works best, is a longer-term recovery plan, that includes treatment as a step-down process involving residential/inpatient, long-term outpatient support, quality mental health care, and vocational training. These are the bare minimums needed for many to be successful. Unfortunately, this may take many years to realize, as the reimbursement system would need to change to accommodate.*

Currently, the reimbursement system is primarily insurance and/or individuals' private pay. Until the insurance industry and the other items, mentioned briefly, are challenged, and changed, we will continue to hear that most people seeking treatment are not going to stay in recovery. To me, that is incredibly sad. I believe the current systems are complicit and are more responsible for those experiencing Substance Use Disorders failure in recovery than the individual themselves.

In closing, I can only add that it has been a pleasure to share my story as it contributes to changes needed with the overall Behavioral Health System/s. In believing, as a Clinical Supervisor, that there is only a mention of Self-Care within our Codes of Ethics, Angela and I firmly believe Self-Care, building resilience, understanding burn-out, collaborating with like-minded people, and providing training for the Supervisee to flourish rather than struggle.

We are doing what we can, where we are, with what we have.

Invitation for Reflection and Action

What are your concerns for the professional development and advancement for your field of practice?

Is there something you can do to help address these concerns?

Who can you ask to join you in this task?

CHAPTER SIX SUMMARY

Peer Collaboration is a requirement of the Licensing Board for Alcohol and Drug Counselors in New Hampshire for license retention. It is one of the built-in mechanisms for accountability to deliver quality services and ultimately protect the public from harm. This is our first ethical call of duty, to do no harm. Elaine Davis and I are extremely fortunate to have found one another in our careers as colleagues in the North Country. It is my hope those of you are starting your careers will discover a colleague who inspires, challenges, and can have fun with you along the way. This is the spirit of Peer Collaboration. The challenges that come with the power differential in the Clinical Supervision relationship need to be explored more especially in the context of how to most effectively support the fastest growing practice in our field right now and that is the peer recovery support worker. This important role presents a paradigm shift out of the traditional clinical model and into what was inspired by the self-help movement with the power of two people working together. Everyone has an important contribution in what is called the continuum of care and everyone deserves equal respect regardless of credential, number of years in sobriety, or whether they experienced an SUD. All experience is valid, and every voice heard. Together Elaine and I hope to contribute value to this discussion.

CHAPTER SIX KEY POINTS

Certified Recovery Support Worker (CRSW)
is the fastest growing SUD Treatment field of practice in New Hampshire.

Leniency bias is the tendency to give undeserving high evaluations on performance evaluations.

Elaine Davis chronicles forty years of SUD treatment in the North Country of New Hampshire.

PART THREE

Advocacy

"I am not sure who it's attributed to,:

**'You have three choices in life, give up,
give in, or give it all you've got.'
Number three has always been my choice."**

Quote contributed by Linda Massimilla
Vice-Chair States and Federal Relations and Veterans Affairs Committee
Grafton 1 New Hampshire State Representative
Find Linda's full Turning Point Story in the Interview Transcripts.

Where Rubber Meets Pavement

This final part of the book is drawn largely from lived experiences and testimony from others on the topic of advocacy ranging from individual activism to the function and role of professional associations and network organizations. It is my hope this material will validate your own experience and inspire you to act in your community, workplace, or within your family and personal relationships.

The evidence is indisputable and continues to mount. The research reviewed in the previous chapters validate the link between clinician well-being, patient care, and safety. Advocating for a work culture inclusive of clinician and worker well-being as an essential component of patient care and safety requires a comprehensive approach involving administration, policy makers, and front-line workers.

The *Quadruple Aim* is a standard of practice model for achieving this by focusing on four targets: public health, reducing costs, quality patient care, and well-being of the care team (Feeley). The *how* of implementing these changes is determined by the work setting and should involve administrative leadership and all workers. This was quickly recognized in the community discussions hosted by the North Country Task Force in its early stages of development.

Although change is inevitable, it is not always easy nor straightforward. Some people seem to be able to roll with that process easier than others. Linda Massimilla is one of those people. I first met Linda prior to her becoming a New Hampshire State Representative and continue to marvel at her ability to engage in important conversations.

She contributed her Turning Point story at the 2018 Best Practices Conference in Waterville Valley, New Hampshire. This event marked the beginning of the North Country Task Force. After reading the update she prepared for this book, I knew it needed to be the introductory story for this final section. If you ever have the pleasure of sharing a conversation with Linda, you will recognize her genuine concern and willingness to do what she can to help, if asked.

More Courageous Conversations.

Linda's 2020 story about becoming a New Hampshire State Legislator.

Find the full transcript of her Turning Point Story in the Interview Transcripts.

Five years ago, I became acutely aware of the drug crisis, when my hometown (population 4,663) had three overdose opioid deaths within a year. Because of our remote North Country location, we had to become resourceful and work collaboratively. In the spring of 2015, concerned about what we, as a community, could do I convened several Substance Use Disorder roundtables made up of physicians and mental health providers, legislators, community outreach and support center personnel, educators, law enforcement, and local elected officials. These meetings morphed into a fall North Country Tri-County Drug Summit that presented nine stakeholder groups with networking opportunities, as well as developing action plans that could be implemented within their communities. In the spring 2016 a follow-up summit was held with a final summit in 2019 that added the compassion fatigue issue. In the summer 2016 I was contacted by a person in recovery who brought to my attention the need for starting another Narcotics Anonymous Group in the area. With her drive and perseverance, we got the first meeting up and running in September. That fall, North Country Health Consortium and I combined forces to present a SUD program and Nar-Can clinic. Although the north country had a residential SUD treatment facility, we had no place for clients to go after they finished their treatment program. In June 2017, a gentleman who had worked in the Substance Use Disorder arena in Massachusetts and was hoping to open recovery housing in the north country was referred to me. After making connections with several community members, civic groups, and faith-based organizations, he opened the first White Mountains Recovery Home in 2017. We now have three more recovery homes in the area illustrating that networking, collaborating, and persevering pay off in the end. I am currently working with a colleague to integrate virtual yoga classes as part of the recovery houses' maintenance program.

Eight years ago, a friend asked me to run for the New Hampshire legislature citing I was well known in the community and the new Hampshire House of Representatives needed more women legislators. As a teacher, I always enjoyed working with and helping people, so I figured this was an opportunity for me to continue doing that. At first, I was tentative because my husband was reluctant about my running, so I offered to run as a write-in. My friend insisted that the only way to possibly be successful would be to file as a candidate, so I did. I will be running for a fifth term in the New Hampshire House this year and grateful for the opportunity I was given to help make a difference.

If people want to make a difference, I advise them to pursue an issue that interests them and/or is passionate about. Participate by taking baby steps, such as volunteering or donating money to an organization that champions their cause. Engage friends and neighbors in discussion groups, write letters to the editor, work for a campaign, run for school board, planning board, selectman, etc. Whatever makes them feel involved.

If you choose a political path, embrace networking opportunities, learn to listen to both sides of the issue, remember that good ideas are not exclusive to one party or group, be willing to compromise, stand up for what you believe, focus on improving, amending or creating new legislation that rights a wrong, improves the human condition, or betters the world.

---

*If you do not know your State Representative,
you can find their contact information by visiting
www.house.gov/representatives/find-your-
representative then type in your zip code.*

*To learn more about what you can do as a citizen
to influence change, contact New Futures 603-225-9540.
www.new-futures.org/our-approach*

In Linda's 2018 Turning Point story she shares the following details about her daily self-care routine: ***What has helped me*** *are the skills I have learned from the alternative therapy courses I have taken. I begin each morning with meridian showers, followed by extending my aura and finally a light exercise. When my life gets hectic and I am feeling tired or stressed, I meditate for fifteen to twenty minutes, which helps bring my life back into focus.*

The Anonymous People

> "Our lives begin to end the day we become
> silent about things that matter."
>
> *Martin Luther King, Jr.*
>
> Quote contributed by Suzanne Thistle, MS, MLADC
> North Country Task Force Policy and Administration Workgroup
> NHADACA Policy Committee Chairperson, 2017-2021
> 2020 Best Selling Author, Chem-Free Sobriety
> Find Sue's full interview in the Turning Point Stories & Interview Transcripts.

CHAPTER SEVEN PREVIEW

The 2013 documentary film *The Anonymous People* is used in this chapter to describe the culture of the 12-step self-help program of Alcoholics Anonymous (A.A.). The title of the film connects A.A. history and tradition with contemporary culture. In doing this, it challenges the A.A. Tradition of anonymity provides a platform for discussing why this is important to the growth of recovery friendly norms in our communities and workplaces.

In the interview with Sue Thistle, she talks about the risks of believing medication is the answer for what ails us and the importance of coming to our own conclusions for what is in our own best interests. *I think Martin Luther King, Jr. says it all. We must stand up for what is right. Pharmaceutical companies want us all to believe that medication is the answer. It is imperative that people understand this. We were deceived about medication with Oxycontin and ACTIQ. Now we must be careful to see how treatment is following the same path. Not all people with an opiate disorder need medication and very few may need it for life. Dr. Amen talks about having a PET scan to help with decision of* *the brain. We cannot just give medicine for a brain disease without knowing how the brain is functioning.*

The Anonymous People

is a feature documentary film produced in 2013 and directed by Greg D. Williams. It is about the 23.5 million Americans living in long-term recovery from alcohol and other drug addiction.

"Anonymity is the spiritual foundation of all our Traditions, ever reminding us to place principles before personalities" ("Understanding Anonymity").

The A.A. Tradition of anonymity reflects the context of our culture here in the United States when this 12-step program was getting started. Prohibition and the Great Depression were in the not too distant past when A.A. began in 1935. In 1951, Al-Anon was established for the family and friends of the Alcoholic and in 1957 Alateen for teenagers struggling with their alcohol use.

The 12-Steps were established as a set of guidelines for spiritual and character development, a blueprint for recovery. These steps continue to serve the same purpose today. It is called a self-help group because the groups are not led by a professional facilitator. It is considered a fellowship without religious affiliation. It is considered a spiritual program by acknowledging the presence of a higher power and allows everyone to define their higher power according to their own understanding.

A.A. had its beginnings in **1935** at Akron, Ohio, as the outcome of a meeting between Bill W., a New York stockbroker, and Dr. Bob S., an Akron surgeon. Both shared the struggle of what is now called an Alcohol Use Disorder ("FAQ").

Privacy and safety are basic building blocks for any trusted relationship. Being able to share our story whether it be with one person or a group of people and doing so without fear of it being used against us at work or in other parts of our lives.

The Eighteenth Amendment was passed by the U.S. Congress in 1917 and illegalized the manufacture, transportation, and sale of alcohol. Nationwide Prohibition lasted from 1920 until 1933 ("How Long Did Prohibition Last?").

Using only first names is another reflection of this tradition. Anonymity was the solution to the challenges of the time, thus Alcoholics Anonymous. Today the program has grown beyond alcohol use, i.e., Overeaters Anonymous, Narcotics Anonymous, Gambling Anonymous, to name a few.

Today, an A.A. presence can be found in approximately 180 nations worldwide, with membership estimated at over two million. There are more than 118,000 A.A. groups around the world and A.A.'s literature has been translated into languages as diverse as Afrikaans, Arabic, Hindi, Nepali, Persian, Swahili, and Vietnamese, among many others ("A.A. Around the World").

In today's culture, stigma, assumptions, and misinformation remain as barriers. The film *Anonymous People* challenges us to examine how not talking openly about the successes of long-term recovery contributes to maintaining these barriers. Conversations on this topic are avoided or minimized therefore inaccurate assumptions, bias, and ill-informed judgments are reinforced because they are not challenged.

The founders of A.A. recorded their stories along with several other founding members in a 575-page volume titled the A.A. Big Book. The first edition was published 1938 with the fourth edition published 2001. It is one of the best-selling books of all time, having sold thirty million copies. In 2011, Time magazine placed the book on its list of the 100 best and most influential books written in English since 1923, the year in which the magazine was first published.

In 2012, the Library of Congress designated it as one of eighty-eight "Books that Shaped America" ("The Big Book"). *The Anonymous People* film honors the legacy of this 12-Step self-help program and celebrates the power of sharing lived-experience through positive messaging.

During the discussion that followed viewing the film, one of the comments stayed with me. The comment referenced the history of non-smoking in public places. I often refer to this when speaking about culture change. In my lifetime, I can remember when it was considered acceptable to smoke while traveling by airplane, while in a restaurant or bar, etc.

The point is cultural norms *can be* changed.

Courageous conversations require feeling safe. Sharing personal experiences without fear of it being used against you is a basic need for building a trusted relationship. At the time, anonymity was the solution and trusting everyone in that sacred circle to leave what was said in that room.

In his interview about how Sober Living Homes cultivate a culture of safety for everyone, Keith Anderson describes the following.

Regarding courageous conversations to reduce stigma that keep people silent about how this work is impacting work-life balance: what practices are you using to create a place for this with your staff & for yourself? *We utilize our managers meetings. All our managers are required to take time off and to take that time away from the homes. We normalize what we go through, many of our managers live in sober houses. So, they are surrounded with questions and situations that arise at any time without expectation. When stress or frustration arises, we are understanding and empathy towards that because who would not get stressed out with those conditions.*

Find Keith's full interview in Turning Point
Stories & Interview Transcripts.

Words are powerful. Choosing our words carefully is important. *The Anonymous People* documentary encourages us to celebrate recovery as a solution to what is currently an incurable chronic disease. It points us in the direction of learning new ways of seeing an old problem and how to craft telling our stories from a thriving and healthy perspective.

Word choices for describing addiction in medical practices has also changed to reflect a more accurate representation of this chronic disease. In 2013, the American Psychological Association updated its language in the 5th revised edition of the Diagnostic Statistical Manual (DSM5).

The DSM5 is the reference manual for medical diagnosis and used for billing purposes. Substance Use Disorder replaced Substance Abuse and Dependence. The new title was chosen as an effort to help "de-stigmatize" a chronic medical condition. Qualifying terms are used to describe severity of the diagnosis, i.e., mild, moderate, severe. Remission and partial remission are used to describe length of time the symptoms of the disorder have not occurred.

Another way to look at this is to consider how other chronic diseases are discussed. Diabetes and cancer do not yet have cures. These are chronic diseases that will get worse without treatment. Symptoms will worsen and lead to death. Treatment of chronic disease without cure is focused on reducing the symptoms. This involves lifestyle changes and developing new habits to support treatment.

Alcoholic or Addict, I believe the original intention of this statement was about accepting responsibility for the behavior contributing to the development of the disease.

The *Anonymous People* film suggests changing this language to something like *"Hello, my name is Angela and I am a person in long term recovery. What this means to me is I have not used alcohol or marijuana in 30 years. This is important to me because I want to be the healthiest best possible me, I can be."*

As part of my recovery plan when preparing for discharge from psychiatric treatment after my plan for suicide, I knew I needed to find a way to speak publicly about my experience. Turns out, the admissions staff on duty when I admitted myself for treatment was also the founder of the local chapter of the National Alliance for Mental Illness (NAMI). This person is also a trainer for the NAMI In Our Own Voices (IOOV) program and provided me with the contact information for these programs near my neighborhood.

People are willing to help, you just need to ask.

The act of following through with making the phone call to connect with my local program came naturally. There are a million reasons we can find to talk ourselves out of something or into something. For example, while writing this book, I have felt twinges of resentment about missing a beautiful day outside or not being part of a movie with my family in the living room. Initially this resentment felt like it was going to cause a problem for me. What has been different, I speak to this feeling—or whatever it is that is distracting me—immediately. My old habits of stubborn independence interfered with me being honest about my needs. I make a different choice and in doing that that choice always has something to do with expressing what is on my mind. So, I have frequent conversations with the people living with me about budgeting my time to do what needs to be done, one day at a time.

Keith Anderson speaks about what he does to maintain his precious 20%:

Regarding the precious 20% of compassion satisfaction: what has your lived experience taught you; what are the "essentials" for you to maintain that precious 20%: *For me personally I must have time to myself. Step work is something that has allowed me to awaken my spirit and keep it awake. However, taking time for a workout in the gym is huge for me. Being in nature, therefore I moved to the mountains in the first place. Taking time with God and being in prayer. Meditation is a valuable tool that I do not get enough of. Being with family is so important. I must allow myself to have time to just disconnect, which is easier said than done.*

Find Keith's full interview in the Turning Point
Stories & Interview Transcripts.

A comment from one of my clients who described their way of "moving forward" that often encourages me to do the same was said something like this *"when I wake up in the morning I get right out of bed because I know if I stay there I will most likely end up procrastinating and my whole day will end up out of kilter."*

Another one...*wake up, get up, make your bed, messy bed, messy head.*

NAMI In Our Own Voice

presentations change attitudes, assumptions, and ideas about people with mental health conditions. These free, 40-, 60-, or 90-minute presentations provide a personal perspective of mental health conditions, as leaders with lived experience talk openly about what it is like to have a mental health condition.

What happened, what helped, what next. Several months later, I completed the IOOV training with eight other people. The training is a group process designed for sharing difficult topics that are deeply personal and designed as a positive messaging campaign to increase awareness and understanding. It is not a therapy group but certainly has a therapeutic effect. We prepared our stories using a format based on three parts; **what happened, what helped, and what next.** Descriptive details are discouraged from being included because this could potentially negatively trigger others. We practiced delivering our stories while in our small groups and then in front of the whole group.

> **In today's context, not talking openly about the successes of long-term recovery contributes to keeping those important courageous conversations silent.**

Up until recent years, most news headlines mentioning a substance use related incident was negative or inflammatory. Journalists like those of the Granite State News Collaborative here in New Hampshire leverage their platform for positive messaging and running stories about solutions rather than sensationalized problems. Choosing to keep our focus on the solution and being willing to learn more about things we think we already know are important when engaging change.

The Granite State News Collaborative

is a statewide multimedia news collaborative that draws on and amplifies the strengths of its members to expand and add missing dimensions to coverage of issues of concern to the New Hampshire public, as well as to communities. Through coordinated reporting and engagement activities, the Collaborative will pursue inclusive and responsive coverage that builds public trust and holds the government accountable to its citizens (Granite State News Collaborative).

Silence and fear cut across all boundaries regardless of the issue or the person involved. Feeling isolated is dangerous while in crisis because it augments fear, insecurity, and often leads to hopelessness. Now with pandemic, data collection is showing an increase in mental health problems associated with social isolation due to quarantine and social distancing ("Quick Covid-19 Primary Care Survey").

> **More than 20 million people in the United States have a substance use disorder.**
>
> **Now, COVID-19 has left many locked down, laid off, and flooded with uncertainty. So far, experts see signs of relapses, rising overdoses, and other worries** (Weiner).

The power of hopelessness draining our will for life is perhaps best described by Viktor Frankl in his first publication Reality Therapy (1949). Frankl's lived experience as a survivor of WWII Nazi Concentration Camps has given us better understanding for what science has proven regarding the significance of our search for meaning.

Contemporary trauma-informed therapies validate Frankl's conclusion: finding and making meaning from tragedy, trauma, or loss is a key factor in recovery and resilience (Masero).

Crisis is opportunity. The pandemic has spurred innovations in addiction treatment, though, and each comes with pluses and minuses. The article *COVID-19 and the opioid crisis: When a pandemic and an epidemic collide* include interviews from across the country to describe how providers and patients are navigating the new normal of pandemic (Weiner).

In regions hit hard by COVID-19 outbreaks, providers quickly moved to provide nearly all care remotely via telehealth platforms. The shift would not have been possible, they say, without the loosening of federal telemedicine rules and payment changes from Medicare and Medicaid. For many patients, the shift online has been a huge help. "Some patients used to have to travel four hours as often as once a week," says Berry.

Calling in is easier than showing up in person in other ways, as well. "Because of the stigma, patients often worry about being seen entering a treatment facility," says Carla Marienfeld, MD, medical director of the University of California San Diego Addiction Recovery and Treatment Program. *"It can be quite intimidating."*

People who have grappled with the lure of drugs say it is a particular hell that only someone else who has gone through it can truly understand. Group sessions with a therapist or a mutual support organization like Narcotics Anonymous, therefore, are frequently crucial to recovery.

Now, many of these groups can only meet over the internet, and patients often miss the in-person connections.

"It's not just the meeting itself," says Quisenberry. *"Before and after the meeting, people would hang out and talk about what has happened to them and what got them through it. You can always learn something that way."* There are also positives to going online, though, including easier access. *"People are able to try out groups that might be further from home but that feel like a really good fit for them,"* Marienfeld says.

Meanwhile, providers in some locations have begun re-initiating in-person group sessions. Still, those will not be quite the same, they note, as participants try to connect behind masks and while sitting six feet apart (Weiner).

In another article published by The Henry J Kaiser Family Foundation in Philadelphia, this description is provided,…*During the pandemic, people taking medication-assisted treatment can renew their prescription every month instead of every week, which helps decrease trips to the pharmacy. It is too soon to know if more people are taking advantage of the new rules, and accessing medication-assisted treatment via telehealth, but if that turns out to be the case, many addiction medicine specialists argue the new rules should become permanent, even after the pandemic ends.*

"If we find that these relaxed restrictions are bringing more people to the table, that presents enormous ethical questions about whether or not the DEA should reinstate these restrictive policies that they had going in the first place," said Dr. Ben Cocchiaro, a physician who treats people with substance use disorder.

Cocchiaro said the whole point of addiction treatment is to facilitate help as soon as someone is ready for it. He hopes if access to recovery can be made simpler during a pandemic, it can remain that way afterward (Feldman).

Invitation for Reflection and Action

If you are not familiar with the 12-step self-help program of Alcoholics Anonymous, check out this website to learn more: www.aa.org/

If you are familiar with the 12-step self-help program, check out SMART Recovery as an additional and alternative resource: www.smartrecovery.org/

Check out the SMART Recovery Toolbox and select the Life Balance Worksheet then complete it. What areas of your life would you like to improve?

Use your SMART goals: **S**pecific
                                      Measurable
                                      Advocate
                                      Relevant
                                      Time-oriented

CHAPTER SEVEN SUMMARY

The self-help movement of Alcoholics Anonymous established a framework that has helped millions of people around the world find another way out of addiction. Our culture has changed, and it is important to adapt to current culture needs as well as to what is helpful to everyone. The chronic disease of addiction is complex. Understanding how the brain functions has allowed us to understand addiction is a neurological disorder. Today we also know the brain can heal itself and we can learn new habits to replace the old unproductive and destructive habits. Many are doing this every day and not all of them are doing this through the 12-step program. The world wide web has increased access to more resources all of which we are learning more about because of having to live with social isolation due to COVID-19. The important message in this chapter is there is more than one pathway of recovery and respecting that individuality must be part of the recovery process. There is always something else to learn.

CHAPTER SEVEN KEY POINTS

The self-help 12-step program Alcoholics Anonymous, began in 1935.

As part of a national effort to more accurately represent this as a chronic disease, the term Substance Use Disorder replaced Substance Abuse and Substance Dependence in the revised edition of the Diagnostic Statistical Manual DSM5(2013).

Positive messaging campaigns such as the documentary film *The Anonymous People* and the *In Our Own Voices* program of the National Alliance for Mental Illness encourage positive culture change.

Practice What You Advocate

> The forces that distract the helper from vigilance can be powerful and persuasive, but we have choices.
>
> If we sort through what's happening, name it, and speak honestly about it, those choices become very clear.
>
> And decisions made in clarity can carry a sort of peace no matter what chaos surrounds us.
>
> *Pamela Woll, 2019*
> *Compassion Doesn't Make You Tired*

CHAPTER EIGHT PREVIEW

This chapter combines lived experiences and expertise of Elizabeth Ropp and her colleague Laura Cooley. Elizabeth is a New Hampshire Licensed Acupuncturist who practices Community Acupuncture and Laura has been involved with National Acupuncture Detoxification Association (NADA) for several decades as a trainer and travels internationally delivering this training.

She recently produced a short DVD titled **Unimagined Bridges,** presenting the history of the NADA 5-point Auricular protocol, its applications, and testimonies from practitioners, researchers, and recipients of its treatment. Their collaboration on changing New Hampshire law to increase access to this service is testimony of how one or two people can create change that helps many. Elizabeth and Laura walk their talk. By the end of this chapter you will have a better understanding of not only how a regular citizen can influence state legislation but also know more about the benefits of the NADA 5-point protocol. Elizabeth and Laura are deep wells of knowledge on this topic therefore, I have included a good bit of direct quotes from their interviews and conversations with me. They are generous with sharing their knowledge and welcome your contact if you wish to learn more from them. You will find their contact information in the biography section toward the back of the book.

Laura's longevity with NADA and experience advocating for legislative support of the NADA protocol has given her insight for effective strategies. This combined with Elizabeth's expertise as a Licensed Acupuncturist made for a successful and swift approach. I should say before going on any further that advocating for legislative change *and* ear acupuncture deserve more attention than this chapter provides. I have included their story as a testimony to how IT IS possible for one or two people to create change that benefits many.

New Hampshire House Bill number 575 (HB 575) was introduced in January 2017 and became law in July 2017 (NH RSA 328-G:9-a). Elizabeth explains in her interview she and Laura worked on the law for seven or eight months. After it became law, there was more work to be done. Elizabeth explained it this way, *Getting the bill passed took nine months from start to finish which included a House Hearing, a subcommittee meeting, a Senate hearing, and a Committee of Conference to remove an terrible amendment. It took an additional twelve months to get the rules passed. The Board of Acupuncture Licensing fought us every step of the way. I attended their board meetings to watch them write the rules and I kept key legislators in the loop. I was a member of the New Hampshire Professional Association at the time. They also opposed the bill. I attended semi-monthly phone meetings. Those meetings were not fun and I dropped my membership with the State Association after that two year time period. I gave myself a lot of ear acupuncture to keep myself calm and to handle the pressure of preparing for hearings or sitting through tense meetings. It turns out the NADA ear acupuncture protocol is exactly what I needed while I was fighting for everyone's right to use it. All of the hard work paid off in the end. **Justice Ruth Bader Ginsberg said it best "You defeat your opponents by outworking them."***

They invested another eighteen months monitoring the rule writing process and a complaint that fought to limit this practice in the rules defined by the New Hampshire Board of Acupuncture. Elizabeth described being on phone meetings regularly with the Acupuncture Professional Association and the Acupuncture Licensing Board and described it as a challenging and difficult process but did not give up, and it paid off in the end.

NH RSA 328-G:9-a allows people who are NADA trained to deliver this ear acupuncture practice to support New Hampshire citizens. Wyoming and Louisiana are the only other states with an equivalent law. The difference between this law and other laws in the United States that people in New Hampshire who have successfully completed the NADA training can treat anyone, anywhere, anytime in New Hampshire. Other states restrict the NADA 5-point protocol to only SUD treatment programs meaning private practice practitioners cannot use it even if NADA trained.

Elizabeth explained, *here in New Hampshire, there are basically two styles for practicing Acupuncture, either in the context of a private room where patients are seen one at a time or seen in the context of a group in a community style setting. The Benefits of social interaction of the community setting have been studied and indicate positive outcomes. The 12-Step Recovery community is an example of the power of a group experience as it has advantages and disadvantages. I refer to my colleague Laura Cooley often when talking about advocacy, Laura says,* **"If you educate legislators well, they quickly do the right thing regardless of who is against it. It all depends on educating them correctly and fully and this involves providing lived experience testimonies."**

Elizabeth goes on to explain "...**one of the most effective ways of doing this is to needle the legislators involved with sponsoring the bill."** Yes, "to needle" means poking needles in their ears! I know, it sounds absurd. Hang in here with me and you will discover how this practice is bringing real-time relief to disaster response teams, emergency first responders, victims of crime and violence, people living with depression, anxiety, and substance use disorders.

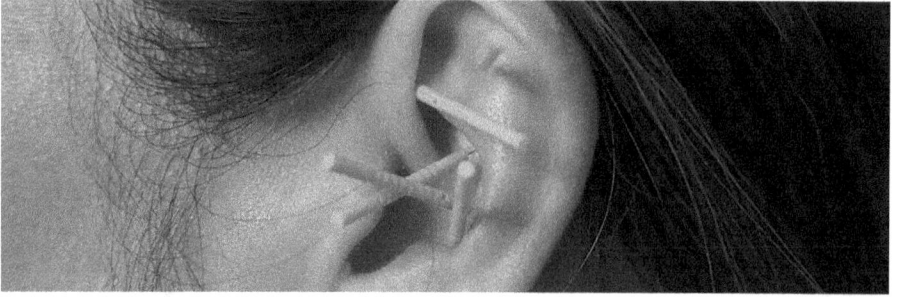

Picture courtesy of trainer Dr. Susana Mendez -Texas

	ORANGE PLASTIC HANDLE EAR ACUPUNCTURE NEEDLE The bright orange handle has been designed for grip and visibility. These were originally used specifically to assist in the detoxification phase of treatment for substance use disorders. The Community Acupuncture model has been applying this safe, simple, and effective tool being used around the world for community wellness, behavioral health, mental health, disaster and emotional trauma. www.acudetox.com/about-nada/

Picture courtesy of trainer Dr. Susana Mendez -Texas

The National Acupuncture Detoxification Association (NADA) is working on public health initiatives to expand access to NADA training and practice for allied health workers.

When describing a successful strategy for getting a law passed, Laura gives New Hampshire Representative Robert Backus the credit for expediting this bill to law. She explained all bills must be presented to the Executive Departments and Administration Committee (EDA). This Committee monitors what can reach the Office of Professional Licensing and Certification.

She said the way Representative Backus introduced his request to pass this bill was simple and direct. Laura described him holding up a letter from the American Acupuncture Council, the largest and oldest insurance company in the United States providing malpractice coverage to Acupuncture practitioners. While doing this, she continued to explain he introduced his expertise as an attorney who handles malpractice suits of lawyers and doctors then calmly stated *the letter is remarkable because it says there are no malpractice claims against an entire class or practitioners—ever—in the thirty-five years the practice has been available in the United States.* Laura explained he ended with a continued calm presentation while explaining he has never seen a letter like this in his career and concluded, "I'm asking you to pass this bill."

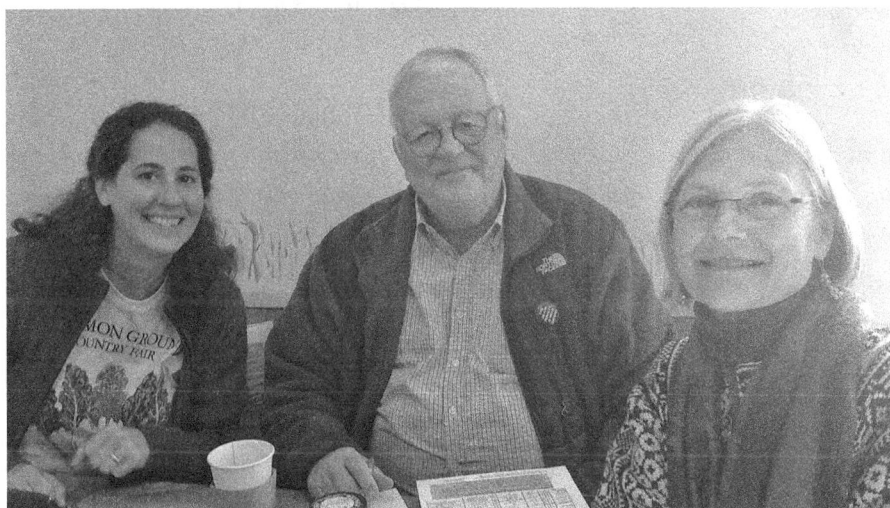

(on the left) Elizabeth Ropp, (center) New Hampshire
Representative Robert "Bob" Backus,
(on the right) Laura Cooley

Eana Meng is a graduate of Harvard University, a historian, and a physician in training.

She has created several historical videos for The Harvard Asia Center.

The word Chi means movement and that means Acupuncture does not DO anything. It is what it allows to happen. It facilitates. It allows flow to restore. It is not a thing. It is movement. All life moves. Every bit of it on every level. Acupuncture restores the flow to coherency. Self-regulation means coherency. When you can self-regulate it means you can bring your nervous system back to coherency. There are many more connections for pleasure in our brain than there are for pain.

Sue Cox demystifies this process of this change. She has trained all of the prison security of the United Kingdom.

The needles are not what you see at the doctor's office. They do not look like traditional acupuncture needles either. The needles used for this 5-point protocol are packaged into a clear sealed envelope not much bigger than a regular size bandage. Five per package. The needle itself looks more like a stiff piece of jewelry wire used for fine beadwork. The needle is mounted into a round plastic rod approximately one inch in length and diameter larger than the lead in a regular pencil. The length of the needle is less than one half of an inch.

On the NADA website this description is found: ***The NADA Protocol is a non-verbal approach to healing. NADA involves the gentle placement of up to five small, sterilized disposable needles into specific sites on each ear.*** www. acudetox.com/nada-protocol/

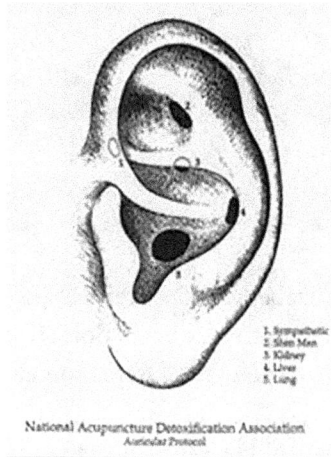

1. Sympathetic
2. Shen Men
3. Kidney
4. Liver
5. Lung

National Acupuncture Detoxification Association
Auricular Protocol

Diagram of the NADA 5-point Auricular
Protocol chart created by Sharon Roos

Prior to the Pandemic, Elizabeth was volunteering her time weekly at Manchester's HOPE Recovery Center in New Hampshire. She and Laura worked together for two years prior advocating for legislative change to increase public access to receiving the 5-point ear acupuncture protocol. As a team, Laura, and Elizabeth's approach to advocating for legislative change confirm one or two people can create positive change for many.

There are twenty accredited Recovery Support Centers in the United States. Seven of those twenty are in New Hampshire.

www.caprss.org/accredited-organizations/

Learn more about Recovery Support Centers in the Resources found in the Action Guide Workbook.

Together and individually, they presented numerous testimonies at New Hampshire Legislative public hearings. Their voices are directly quoted throughout this chapter. Elizabeth explains the differences between a Community Acupuncturist and a Private Acupuncturist. What is more, she describes her own experience with stress response symptoms at that time and how she established a safe and easy self-treatment using the 5-point protocol.

The National Acupuncture Detoxification Association (NADA) protocol was originally used as a supportive component in drug and alcohol treatment settings. It used a 3-5 point ear acupuncture formula to ease withdrawal symptoms and helped patients become more clear-headed and comfortable.

The NADA Protocol is a non-verbal approach to healing and involves the gentle placement of up to five small, sterilized disposable needles into specific sites on each ear. It was first developed in the 1970s at Lincoln Hospital in the Bronx, New York.

It can be easily used in any location where a group of people can sit together. It is most commonly used for addictions, behavioral health, disasters, and emotional trauma. It is a technique that is versatile, effective, and economical.

A variety of Healthcare Practitioners and Community Members have been trained as Auricular Detox Specialists (ADS) including addiction workers, acupuncturists, community health workers, social workers, and family members. www.acudetox.com/

Stuyt, Elizabeth, and Claudia Voyles. "The National Acupuncture Detoxification Association protocol, auricular acupuncture to support patients with substance abuse and behavioral health disorders: current perspectives." *Substance Abuse and Rehabilitation,* vol. 7, pp. 169-180, 2016, doi: 10.2147/SAR.S99161.

Find more related articles in the Resources in the Action Guide Workbook.

In her interview with me, **Elizabeth describes the stress response symptoms she began experiencing** during the two years of her work with the legislators. Her experience is testimony of how the stress response can also happen with positive events rather than a negative trauma or adverse experience. In this portion of the interview she is describing her collaboration with the New Hampshire legislator who sponsored the bill she and Laura were successful at getting passed.

Find Elizabeth's full interview in the Transcripts.

The work took its toll on me. I was fighting so hard. It began to spill over into other areas of my life and home. My husband was between jobs at the time, so he was available. I was in the kitchen...he said, "You are steamrolling." When my husband said this, I was haphazardly pushing things out of the way in the kitchen. I realized then I was angry and overwhelmed but also filled with inspiration and feeling totally in the moment...it was the first time in my life the mind chatter was not in my life...I felt so completely focused.

Huck gave me a strategy to have all different kinds of people testify and speak to different aspects of why this bill needs to pass. My initial strategy was to ask my patients to call their legislator...that, plus showing up to the Acupuncture Professional Association meetings. They gave me a minute to speak, one who had been a thorn in my side then started yelling at me and criticizing me saying awful things...it was awful.

2017 somatic symptoms started early winter fight flight state "panic".

*I lost my appetite, I had a hard time sleeping, difficulty focusing, and wanted to run in different directions...my husband tried to help me and said we need to sit down and work through this one thing at a time...**That's when I started treating myself with the 5-point ear protocol for 20 minutes a day.** That is all I needed to do to get myself focused and move forward. When my anxiety was so bad, I treated myself with the NADA protocol 2-3 times a day. A 20-minute treatment was usually enough to keep me focused and grounded.*

***In January 2018,** I attended by conference call, the New Hampshire Acupuncture Board meetings. I was also working 20-25 hours per week at the clinic. I would get home and work on the computer or phone to get the bill a number. You do not know when your hearing is going to happen, you must check every day—I did this for four-weeks. **You must check the website every week, on Thursdays.** It finally said the hearing would be on Valentine's day. I had about two weeks to get people together to testify. My husband helped me a lot. He became my communications proofreader...it was like a crazy magical time.*

Elizabeth's ability to recognize her own stress response enabled her to practice what she and Laura advocate. Her testimony is a living example of how we can engage our stress response through conscious choice rather than allowing ourselves to be swept into panic or other maladaptive responses.

The phrase Jon Kabat Zinn uses to describe the purpose for learning these techniques sums this up best. (the creator of Mindfulness Based Stress Reduction)

You can't stop the waves, but you can learn to surf.

In her interview, Elizabeth describes the benefits of the self-care practice she established during that very busy time in her career: How are your symptoms now—You described them at their worst winter 2017. *Now much better, I am not in that hectic place anymore. I have worked on other bills. Now that I have done it and know what I'm doing. I am not as stressed. But also, I feel like I already got the most important bill passed. I've never experienced stress that intense before. It lasted for so many weeks...living with all those deadlines...I still give myself ear acupuncture treatments as a prep...now I love going to the state house. Laura and I put two years of time providing free acupuncture at the State House. The committee knows us now.*

How do you explain the mechanism of change in the 5 points in the ear? *Laura Cooley and I have talked a lot about this.*

It is more about what the ear acupuncture allows to happen, rather than what it does for you. *Dr. Tom Corbin explains this as part of Vagal nerve stimulation. Needling points in the ear. This is close to the ear canal. This is stimulating the Vagal nerve and gets people out of the fight or flight mode. Dry mouth is a signal of fight or flight mode. I had that a lot when I was speaking before the Board and the Legislators.*

In **Unimagined Bridges**, Laura uses the term AcuReSet to describe this practice because it serves beyond the needs of treating addiction and describes this as "resetting the stress response to relax..." In this summary of the NADA 5-point Protocol, its origins, and more recent applications to first responders at ground zero after the terrorist attacks on the Twin Towers in New York City. She described a moving testimony delivered by the president of the Louisiana Firefighters Union at the 2010 NADA conference held in New Orleans that year. She said while he was describing their experience of receiving this care, he teared up and said he "didn't know what he would have done if these resources hadn't been available."

In Laura's words for describing the back scene to this story, *The guys convinced him to get treatment right in the middle of it all, maybe three weeks in, and he went to sleep for four hours. That's why the International Fire Fighters flew*

Wendy and the three massage therapists she was with, from Baton Rouge to the Command Post in NOLA, where they were for three weeks.

Our conference was in 2010 in New Orleans. Chad Major, President of Professional Fire Fighters of Louisiana (PFFL) was the speaker at the NADA Conference. The Command Post in Baton Rouge was a Church, where firefighters, others that had responded, Wendy and the 3 massage therapists were brought to once they got to Los Angeles. The guys were other firefighters who had already had treatment. The one Massage therapist has a company providing corporate Wellness, and she had a contract with HBO. Wendy provided acupuncture every Friday at HBO for years. HBO mounted a response to Katrina, offering them vaccines for going into a disaster zone. Wendy worked at the Fire Department at that time and her supervisor told her if she even thought about going down to Katrina, she wouldn't have a job—and she did lose her job—that's the way I remember it (her supervisor appeared to dislike her, I can attest to the venom she spewed in my direction about Wendy, knowing I was her colleague and friend). Those who found and established successful programs are frequently targeted by others.

Chad Major was also the firefighter's lobbyist and was of major assistance in getting the LA legislature to vote unanimously the NADA bill into law, which also got licensed acupuncturists out from under a requirement that to practice they had to be employed by a physician, which none of the eleven in the state were. I literally have a letter from the NOFD supporting the deregulation of acupuncturists via this law so they could practice freely, and acupuncture would be more accessible to firefighters. I have the letter— last I looked and there are over 60 there now. Wendy and that team went to Baton Rouge in mid- September, 2005.

She had an invitation extended by a Search and Rescue organization. One needs a formal letter of invitation to get through in a disaster zone. Marc O'Regan, a Navy Seal, boat operator, acupuncturist, PA, massage therapist was the only one that could respond to the directions to go to Baltimore airport and wait for instructions. Mark O'Regan was the first of our team in the disaster zone, and he only massaged people, telling me he saw his job as helping people with immediate needs and giving massages, so that when we arrived we would be welcomed. He did not feel it was time yet to propose needles.

Once Chad Major had his 4 hour nap, the International Association of Fire Fighters put them on a little plane and flew them into New Orleans (NOLA) to be on the Command post, where all fire and EMS services were being run out of—and fortunately was within walking distance of my aunt and uncle's *house, my uncle actually taught at Holy Cross, where the Command Post was. All the Irish visiting firefighters stole all the crucifixes in the place!*

Wendy is co-founder of CRREW (Community Relief and Rebuilding Through Education & Wellness), *and the NADA trainer that got acupuncture into the New York City Fire Department via grant funding and served the fire houses for some time, a grassroots project supplying equipment to rescue and recovery workers at ground zero would indicate what firehouses might need support and give their contact information, then developing a flexible team of volunteers that could roll with the unexpected, which might mean when you show up at the agreed time and your services are turned away or the house is on a call and there is no one to treat. If an acupuncturist wanted to work in firehouses, she would find out where they live, where they work, a firehouse on her route, go there and start feeding the dog treats till the House would be open to the idea. The Grant provided funding for NADA and a full body at the five counseling centers, volunteers served individual firehouses, we would attend the Firehouse picnics, which all Firehouses in NYC do annually, and their holidays parties. Wendy set up a juicing bar, ear acupuncture, massage, crafts for kids, herbal and dietary advice—it was a blast! Loved it as I would go down and do the picnics, etc., with her, she had just about finished her acupuncture training when 9/11 hit, but NADA trained, she organized and treated a whole lot of people.*

She got through three levels of security without credentials to be on site at ground zero in the FEMA trailer to do ear acupuncture there on firefighters taking a break from the digging.

I will finish with the quote Danny Adams gave to me. He and Chad Major are tight, they have been there since Katrina and are still there. Danny Adams is the First Responder Coordinator for the Louisiana Spirit Coastal Counseling Program.

"Since 2005 I have had the opportunity to see for myself the effects of the Acudetox method of acupuncture on first responders in Louisiana. Doing CISM and outreach to first responders after disasters is incredibly difficult to do, but with acupuncture I have seen first responders be still and quiet for a short period to relax for a change. During this we have an open window of opportunity to get first responders back on track with their objectives they are assigned to do. We found better sleep and less frustration as a result of acupuncture with first responders. In a real true effort, I would love to see the acupuncturist model on a national basis to outreach to first responders. I see less suicides, divorce rates, addictive disorders, and abuse because of working together."

Find Laura's full interview in the Transcripts.

In New Hampshire, we are fortunate to have an organization dedicated to policy development and change. On their website www.new-futures.org/ it says, *New Futures is a nonpartisan, nonprofit organization that advocates, educates, and collaborates to improve the health and wellness of all New Hampshire residents through policy change.*

New Futures offer technical support and training for New Hampshire citizens and organizations wanting to make a difference on issues of concern. Additional resources are available in the Resource section of the Action Guide Workbook.

CHAPTER EIGHT SUMMARY

Any kind of change requires motivation. In terms of advocating for policy change or changes in law, being motivated is not enough. A coordinated effort is required. Laura and Elizabeth's experience illustrates the involvement and commitment required to create policy change. More importantly, about promoting self-care, Elizabeth's testimony confirms we can also experience *negative effects* like what she experienced, nausea, headaches, body aches, and interrupted sleep. Although Elizabeth's involvement in this task is clearly a part of what defines her precious 20% of compassion satisfaction, her body began telling her when things began to get out of balance. Fortunately, for her, she had the insight and understanding to listen to the signals her body was generating and responded in a way that helped her re-establish balance by applying the treatment she gives to others to herself. This is just like what flight attendants instruct us to do in the event of an emergency;

"Put your oxygen mask on first, then help others".

Her story shows us that our personal self-care is an everyday necessity and not just for when we are tired, frustrated, or unhappy. Getting involved with changing policy and law are possible when combining strategic communications, community engagement, and subject matter expertise. This three-pronged approach to legislative change described by Laura and Elizabeth's experience is the model used by New Futures in New Hampshire. New

Futures provide the technical assistance and training for how to engage advocacy and campaigning for change. Find New Futures contact information in the Resource section. Laura and Elizabeth's contact information are also found in the biography section of the book.

Invitation for Reflection and Action

Think about a time you experienced physical symptoms associated with work related stress.

How frequent do/did these symptoms occur?

What helped you get through that difficult time?

Listen to an interview of Laura Cooley and Elizabeth Ropp describing the NADA 5-point ear acupuncture protocol and the history behind its development

www.asiacenter.harvard.edu/announcements/new-video-release-its-first-aid-tracing-global-transmission-five-point-ear

---

Leadership and the Role of Network Organizations

> "We cannot solve problems with the same
> thinking we used to create them."
>
> *Albert Einstein*

Quote contributed by Dr. Sally Garhart, MD
Find her contribution to the Turning Point Stories in the Interview Transcripts.

CHAPTER NINE PREVIEW

This final chapter summarizes what began as a private conversation and quickly became part of a national movement. The *Quadruple Aim* is briefly reviewed as the model for work culture standards inclusive of clinician well-being as a norm for delivering quality patient and client care. Interviews with my New Hampshire colleagues provide practical advice and clear direction for how individuals are creating these important changes in their unique workplace culture. The ethical standards of practice for addiction professionals are reviewed. These ethical principles reinforce pre-existing evidence identifying self-care as an ethical imperative to quality patient care and safe delivery of treatment services. Detailed instructions are included from the National Academy of Medicine (NAM) Action Collaborative for Clinician Well-Being and Resilience for how to become a Network Organization. Submitting a Commitment Statement to the NAM Action Collaborative is the only requirement for becoming a Network Organizations. No fees are involved, it is free.

The Commitment Statement from the New Hampshire Alcohol and Drug Abuse Counselors Association is also included with a chronological review of the process leading up to NHADACA becoming the first organization in New Hampshire to join this national movement.

It all began with the release of the 1999 landmark report *To Err is Human.* This report revealed that many hospital deaths are due to errors. For those of us who consider reading academic and scientific research reports not part of our repertoire of leisure reading and prefer "seeing the movie", the 2019 documentary film is now available (*To Err is Human*).

This Mission Statement is posted on the homepage of the film's website:

Medical mistakes lead to as many as 440,000 preventable
deaths every year, making it the
#3 leading cause of death in the United States.

To Err is Human is an in-depth documentary about this silent epidemic
and those working quietly behind the scenes to fix it.

We created this film to showcase solutions that are easy to implement
and would dramatically improve the quality of healthcare immediately.

While access to care is a vital flashpoint in
America right now, it is equally
important to ensure the quality of that care is improving, and
not actually causing unnecessary harm or death.

The documentary focuses on the idea of a
new culture of safety in medicine
through the efforts of a select few who believe the system can improve
first acknowledging its imperfections.

Mike Eisenberg directed the film and says; *This topic in particular holds a personal connection to me as the son of patient safety pioneer, the late Dr. John M. Eisenberg. Before he passed away in 2002, my father's work in this field led to a national discussion on medical mistakes and he was the driving force behind* *federal efforts to improve patient safety. Through this film, we hope to carry on his legacy by providing a productive look at the healthcare quality today and how we can do better, rather than a "gotcha" documentary. Those who work in healthcare today want to help patients, but sometimes the system is designed in a way that prevents them from doing just that.*

You will find quite a few short YouTube recordings of interviews with Mike Eisenberg about this film and the meaning it brings to the global discussion on the topic of healthcare. I watched the film and found its impact like how I previously described after watching the documentary *The Anonymous People.* It was profoundly validating and a game changer for my thinking about what difference it makes if I care or not about these things. **Inspiration to do what is necessary to NOT be too tired to care.**

As human beings, we are empathetic creatures and sharing our story matters. Research Professor at Houston, Texas, whose favorite shoes are cowgirl boots (and, by the way, one of my heroes) now New York Times Best Seller Brené Brown says it best,

> *I believe that you have to walk through*
> *vulnerability to get to courage, therefore,*

> ***...embrace the suck.***

That 1999 landmark report jump-started more research and more studies and more reports. Thanks to the people who enjoy that and are great at it, we now have an enormous amount of validated evidence pointing us in the direction we need to be going with our healthcare system. It is up to each of us to help move this process in that direction and the way we do that is going to depend on the work culture of our setting. The sources I have found most relevant to my practice and with my colleagues in my neck of the woods are the National Academy of Medicine's Action Collaborative for Clinician Well-Being and Resilience and the *Quadruple Aim.*

The *Quadruple Aim* concept has been around for a while. It began as the *Triple Aim* in 2007 and was introduced by the Institute for Healthcare Improvement during a fierce debate over reforming health care in the United States. The goal: to provide a framework for a health care system focused not on volume, but on improved quality and patient satisfaction, better outcomes, and reduced costs (Berwick).

Over time, the *Triple Aim* became more than a concept. In the health care world, it is the foundation of everything from laws to strategic plans. It has been tested by the realities of the healthcare environment. Like most things, there is a need to grow and adapt over time. Although the focus on better outcomes, improved care, and lower costs is still fundamental, increasing administrative, regulatory, and professional burdens are leading to clinician burnout and running counter to the goals of the triple aim. This has led to a call for a fourth aim addressing professional well-being.

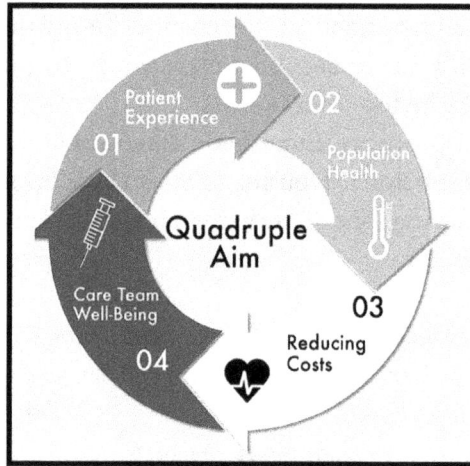

(illustration) www.dapasoft.com/quadruple-aim-role-digitization-ohts/

More importantly, the *Quadruple Aim* is an internationally recognized validation of self-care as a standard of practice.

The World Health Organization has also validated this by announcing their definition of burnout as an "occupational phenomenon due to unsuccessful management of chronic workplace stress."

The solution is a shared responsibility among all of us as workers, employers, supervisors, managers, administrators, corporate executive officers, citizens, and legislators.

Although the *Quadruple Aim* is a comprehensive model designed for the primary care practice and hospital setting, the basic principles involving work-life balance are applicable to all human service work settings.

The backbone of any effective health care system is an engaged and productive workforce, and members of the health care workforce have reported widespread burnout and dissatisfaction. Burnout among the health care workforce can threaten the success of *Triple Aim* by lowering patient satisfaction and increasing the possibility of errors (Bodenheimer). Caregiver burnout among nurses and other team members may contribute to the overuse of resources and increased costs of care (Itchhaporia).

Professional burnout is characterized by loss of enthusiasm for work, feelings of cynicism and a low sense of personal accomplishment, and is associated with early retirement, alcohol use, and suicidal ideation. According to a 2013 RAND Corporation survey , the principal driver of physician satisfaction is the ability to provide quality care (Friedberg). Again, I say, all of this also applies to behavioral health and substance use disorder treatment providers.

The American College of Cardiology (ACC) President C. Michael Valentine, MD, addresses the *Quadruple Aim* and the importance of professional well-being in his 2018 article "Tackling the Quadruple Aim: Helping Cardiovascular Professionals Find Work-Life Balance," published in the *Journal of the American College of Cardiology*. He says,

"For the majority of physicians, we practice medicine because of our passion for improving and saving the lives of patients."

"We can and must take care of ourselves to best take care of those we took an oath to serve"(Valentine).

This is where all of us, regardless of our training or work setting, share common ground.

We do what we do because we love doing it.

Our capacity for empathy and ability to communicate this in the delivery of our professional service is often referred to as "bedside manner". Although this term is associated with hospital work culture, I have often heard it used in other settings. This empathetic capacity, our bedside manner, is also the very thing that can exhaust us, thus the term compassion fatigue. Knowing how to gauge our giving, temper our passion, and practice self-care are important skills for managing our capacity to care.

The four-steps of HomeBase are an easy evidence-informed method to practice self-care anytime and anywhere. Now is an invitation to let yourself try it out for the first time or practice what you already know.

Feet Flat on the Floor
Long Spine
Relaxed Throat
Soft Jaw

Breathe 6 Rounds
One round = inhale and exhale
2x exhale
Your exhale is twice as long as your inhale

Allow your breathing to be relaxed. Do not push yourself. Return to your "normal" breath pattern if you begin to feel uneasy, dizzy, anxious, or uncomfortable. Just like with any new skill, practice takes time, and in time, with practice, it gets easier. Be patient with yourself.

The term compassion fatigue has been used so much in my work culture that many of us are tired of hearing it. I think Pamela Woll does a beautiful job addressing this term in her 2019 book "Compassion doesn't make you tired".

...beware the term "compassion fatigue." Not only is it wobbly, but it's also a catch-all term. There are several conditions whose signs or symptoms overlap with those attributed to compassion fatigue. These are conditions that people might own and address much sooner if they didn't pounce on "compassion fatigue" as the explanation.

If you're "diagnosed" with compassion fatigue—or if you just want to avoid it—most of the advice you'll get will be generic, positive, helpful: Take some time off, build a support network, join a gym, take a bubble bath. But that advice may also be a bit of a tease, especially if you're carrying a bottomless caseload, pulling down double shifts, or topping off a full-time job with all-night caregiving.

Who has time for a bubble bath? But what if there's something else going on, but instead of searching your experience for a deeper understanding, you stop digging at "compassion fatigue"? With that catch-all term as your explanation, you might limit your efforts to standard stress-management techniques. Those tech-

niques may be positive, even important, but they won't address many of the conditions that might be behind your current challenges.

The term moral injury was introduced earlier in the book and originally used to describe the impact of war on combat veterans. I have had the honor of sitting with a combat veteran to hear their story. My role was to help them remain on a path of recovery from the effects of moral injury. Although I had read about moral injury and have specialized training in trauma-sensitive practices, this soldier taught me its meaning. This understanding isn't just about hearing the words spoken, but also being in that moment with the tone and spirit of how they spoke the words describing their experience. I cannot recreate that moment writing about it, but I can share a description.

First, understand a soldier's call to duty and code of honor is to protect and to serve. The bottom line for military and public safety training is learning how to kill another human being. Casualties are the outcome of war. Second, understand that following orders from the command officer is part of the code of honor. Now, imagine you are a soldier, your directive is to secure a designated area from all threats. In this situation, the "enemy" did not wear identifiable uniforms, so everyone, other than your team, could be a threat. You identify a possible threat and receive confirmation the target is a real threat; however, the target is using a child as a shield. To eliminate the threat, you must also shoot the child. Not to eliminate the threat is a dishonorable act that could result in loss of all military benefits for you and your family. This soldier followed orders, eliminated the threat, accomplished the order, and the child was killed. This soldier received honorable recognition and returned home safe but couldn't sleep and experienced other problematic symptoms because of all that you can imagine that would come with being responsible for the death of an innocent child.

This is the essence of a moral dilemma: two conflicting "rights". A trivial example to demonstrate the opposite end of the intensity factor in day-to-day dilemmas is to think of the times you have been faced with two not so great or lousy choices where a decision needed to be made. Did you ever say to yourself, "Well, I'll do the lesser of the two evils"? In the case of a moral injury, there is no lesser evil.

I was attending a seminar on moral injury when I heard the best description I've ever read or heard regarding the difference between post-traumatic stress and moral injury. The presenter was part of a group of veterans who volunteer their time at events like this one to educate others about their experience in recovery from moral injury and the traumas of war. This veteran described both involve soul wrenching pain and said,

> **"This moral injury is from what I've done and the trauma stuff is what happened to me and around me."**

Moral injury is now being used to describe the type of burnout many healthcare professionals are experiencing. Dr. Valentine's words illuminate some of the sources of this dilemma, the competing directives of financial obligations and our ethical duty to first do no harm in the delivery of our care.

Causes of burnout on a broad scale include too many regulations, computerization of practices, number of hours worked, health care reform laws, and lack of professional fulfillment, lack of work-life balance, maintenance of certification (MOC), reimbursement challenges, electronic health record challenges that take away from patient time, prior authorization, and quality reporting among the top issues keeping them up at night (Lewis). Additionally, the shift from private practice to hospital ownership or integration has left many cardiologists frustrated and feeling underappreciated with little options for recourse.

This naming of competing priorities helped me see my circumstances were not an isolated anomaly but rather part of a growing trend across the country. The more I read the research associated with the *Quadruple Aim* the more I could see how the work-life balance equation includes the function of the system. When I dug into my immediate resources for a point of reference, this grabbed my attention in the Code of Ethics published by the National Association for Drug and Alcohol Counselors as if I had never seen it before. You know, one of those experiences when you realize you've been looking at something but not "seeing" it.

National Association for Alcohol and Drug Abuse Counselors
Code of Ethics
Principle VIII-9 Crossroads (NAADAC)

Addiction Professionals may find themselves at a crossroads

when the demands of an organization where the Provider is affiliated poses a conflict with the NAADAC Code of Ethics. Providers shall determine the nature of the conflict and shall discuss the conflict with their supervisor or other relevant person at the organization in question, expressing their commitment to the NAADAC Code of Ethics. Providers shall attempt to work through the appropriate channels to address the concern.

This definition of crossroads rang true for me. I found myself, along with many of my colleagues in New Hampshire, at a crossroads. Practice compromised because our workforce did not and is still struggling with a shortage of qualified workers to meet treatment demands. So we were, and still are, doing the best we can with what we have. Everyone working in good faith to minimize risks to quality care and most importantly patient safety.

As a soldier has a duty and a code of honor, so do we, as healers and helpers and that is to first, do no harm.

This topic of ethical and moral dilemmas during times of crisis is beyond the scope of this book. The point I want to make is this, our code of ethics (as addiction professionals), as is with all professional practices, anticipates these tough spots and are there to clear the fog when things get muddled. As Mike Einsenberg said about his intention for producing the documentary about *To Err is Human*, "this discussion isn't about 'gotcha,'" or who is to blame but rather how we can help each other find a better way so everyone involved is served a win-win.

The *Quadruple Aim* is a compass for achieving more effective work culture environments (Bodenheimer). This information and the material being circulated by the Action Collaborative for Clinician Well-Being and Resilience at the National Academy of Medicine gave me the resources I needed to move beyond my faulty thinking and lack of serotonin, endorphins, and dopamine, all the feel good hormones. My out of whack life-work balance lead me to thinking the lesser of the two evils in my circumstances was to end my life by suicide. Up until then, I believed I was a survivor having survived some pretty tough stuff and always came out on the other side stronger. You know, "What doesn't kill ya makes ya stronger" kind of thinking. At the time, I felt like I had failed at fixing anything. I no longer felt effective. My compassion satisfaction meter had dropped well below that precious 20%. I was too tired to care.

At the time, I was employed as the licensed Clinical Director of a long-time established multi-level of care addiction treatment center. The prior year, the U.S. Surgeon General announced Addiction as a National Epidemic.

Resources and funding were being leveraged but New Hampshire had been feeling the impact of this epidemic long before the Surgeon General published his 2016 report. The workforce in the entire state had been struggling to keep up with the demand for care. One of the responsibilities as the licensed Clinical Director includes signing off on the insurance claims to receive payment. This is a standard of practice designed as an assurance for quality care and means the license holder assumes legal responsibility for the services delivered. Most staff were not yet credentialled and our training program could not go fast enough to keep up with the demand of care.

Complaints were coming in from staff and family members of our clients. Soon afterwards, a client in the residential program overdosed with an unprescribed medication during evening hours. Fortunately, the evening shift staff had recently completed the Narcan training and knew what to do. The following week, another residential client attempted suicide. No one was fatally injured, and the two individuals were transferred to treatment facilities where their medical needs could be treated. I was already feeling like I was in a sinking boat, but this was like boulders being tossed in with me.

The life part of my work-life balance had been out of whack for many months. My family was experiencing significant life transitions. I had already taken two medical leaves of absence to assist my ailing parents. Then my mother died after a courageous battle with cancer. I am grateful to have had the time to be with her and my family through it all. Burning the candle at both ends isn't meant to be a long-term strategy. I was exhausted. I needed to make a choice.

I'm lucky to have had colleagues around me to help me navigate those days. You have met most of these colleagues in the previous chapters. It also seemed lucky that we found a replacement for the Clinical Director position soon after I submitted my resignation. Together we worked with the management team to establish a corrective action plan to address and resolve the complaints and compliance issues. Walking away from that job was easier knowing I was not leaving a sinking boat behind. The treatment center has since gone through many positive changes and now part of a comprehensive community health care system.

The case examples reviewed in the body of work contributing to the *Quadruple Aim* model reflect the hallmarks of the experience I just described and are familiar to many. In time, with more courageous conversations, the principles of this model will take root in behavioral health and substance use disorder fields of practice. The New HampshireBureau of Drug and Alcohol Services has been promoting treatment across the continuum for years (Continuum).

Crisis is pushing us to do what science and research has already been saying we need to do.

In the presentation to his professional group, Dr. Valentine announced the following,

*The ACC has joined the **Academy of Medicine Action Collaborative** in formally committing to promote clinician well-being and combat burnout. More than 130 organizations are part of this collaborative, which aims to support clinician well-being through sustained attention and action at the organizational, state, and national levels, as well as investment in research and information-sharing to advance evidence-based solutions. The ACC is proud to be a part of this effort and is fully committed to helping its members find, implement, and share innovative solutions to burnout, attrition, and poor team functioning.*

About the Clinician Well-Being Collaborative

In 2017, the National Academy of Medicine launched the Action Collaborative on Clinician Well-Being and Resilience, a network of more than 200 organizations committed to reversing trends in clinician burnout . The Collaborative has three goals:

1. *Raise the visibility of clinician anxiety, burnout, depression, stress, and suicide*
2. *Improve baseline understanding of challenges to clinician well-being*
3. *Advance evidence-based, multidisciplinary solutions to improve patient care by caring for the caregiver.*

The Action Collaborative will meet over the course of four years to identify evidence-based strategies to improve clinician well-being at both the individual and systems levels. Products and activities of the Action Collaborative include an online knowledge hub, a series of NAM Perspectives discussion papers, and an all-encompassing conceptual model that reflects the domains affecting clinician well-being. Questions? Contact us at ClinicianWellBeing@nas.edu.

Change begins with one step. In this case, individual, private, courageous conversations initiated a small grassroots movement that became the North Country Task Force. Momentum from that effort quickly found alignment with the goals of the National Academy of Medicine's National Call to Action for Clinician Well-Being and Resilience.

The work initiated by the Task Force evolved into five different work groups each with unique focus on their specific work culture. The Mission and Vision of the New Hampshire Alcohol and Drug Abuse Counselors Association (NHADACA) aligned well with the Task Force Health Care Work Group and timing has been right for this collaboration.

Self-care ethical standards of practice for Substance Use Disorder professionals are found in three out of the nine principles published by the National Association for Alcohol and Drug Abuse Counselors. The impact of the ongoing burden of treatment needs constantly being greater than our workforce capacity has made it clear our focus must include how to support building a resilient and sustainable workforce.

Principles I: The Counseling Relationship
Principle II: Confidentiality and Privileged Communication
Principle III: Professional Responsibilities and Workplace Standards
Principle IV: Working in A Culturally-Diverse World
Principle V: Assessment, Evaluation and Interpretation
Principle VI: E-Therapy, E-Supervision and Social Media
Principle VII: Supervision and Consultation
Principle VIII: Resolving Ethical Concerns
Principle IX: Publication and Communications

Self-care principles

Principle III. Professional Responsibility and Workplace Standards

> **III-18. Self-Monitoring.**...are continuously self-monitoring in order to meet their professional obligations....shall engage in activities that promote and maintain their physical, psychological, emotional, and spiritual well-being.

III-41. Impairment....shall recognize the effect of impairment on professional performance and shall seek appropriate professional...for any personal problems...that may impair work performance or clinical judgement....shall continuously monitor...for signs of impairment... abide by statutory mandates specific to professional impairment when addressing one's own impairment.

Principle VII: Supervision and Consultation

VII: 17. Impairment. Supervisees, including interns and students, shall monitor themselves for signs of physical, psychological, and/or emotional impairment....shall notify their institutional program of the impairment and shall seek appropriate guidance and assistance.

Self-monitoring for impairment of ourselves and each other is written in various ways in these principles. Remember the outcomes of the provider needs assessment presented earlier? 96% of the respondents met at risk criteria for compassion fatigue and burnout. Nearly half reported they weren't talking about these symptoms in their supervision and the remaining reported not having any supervision at all.

The question about impairment and how to evaluate it was explored in the first part of the book. The American Psychological Association has invested a great deal of time addressing this question. In their 2006 report ADVANCING COLLEAGUE ASSISTANCE IN PROFESSIONAL PSYCHOLOGY they present a comprehensive examination of these challenges. Updates on this topic are regularly posted on their website. They say this about impairment. *Impairment therefore refers to circumstances where professional ability is compromised...Impairment, while heightening the risk for ethical violations, does not infer such violations....*

These words help ease the fear about impairment without implying leniency bias. I call this compassionate accountability without shaming or humiliation. In the 2006 report, the stress-distress-impairment continuum is defined. I've translated it into the below illustration to make it easier to understand. I refer to this image frequently with the folks I supervise and have found this helps break the ice around talking about impairment. When people begin to feel safe with their vulnerability, courageous conversations are possible.

Stress – Distress - Continuum

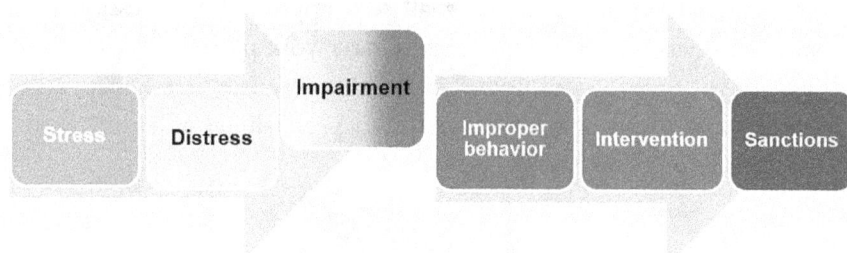

Supervision and Peer Collaboration, as discussed earlier, are basic risk management mechanisms built into our system that are not being effectively utilized. The World Health Organization acknowledges this in their 2019 revised definition of burnout, "an occupational phenomenon due to unsuccessfully managed chronic workplace stress."

The final reference I will make regarding ethical codes of practice from NAADAC Principle VII: Supervision and Consultation - 24 Current practices....*shall ensure…program content and instruction are based on the most current knowledge and information available in the profession....*

As a licensed clinical supervisor, I have witnessed firsthand the standards of practice for supervision are in need of an upgrade in order to keep up with the needs of current times. In chapter six, the work Elaine Davis and I are doing with the help of the North Country Serenity Center in Littleton and the Family Resource Center in Gorham, was introduced. We are working with a great group of people who are doing important work in our communities as Recovery Support Workers.

These folks are on the front lines, doing home visits, helping parents achieve reunification with their children, assisting with the transition from incarceration into a sober living environment, preparing resumes, finding employment, connecting with healthcare, etc. Without their dedicated work, many would never be introduced to recovery and without opportunity, there is no progress, and no change.

This is testimony for how a small community can be an advantage and a strength when a common goal is identified among a few determined and committed citizens. **In Chapter Three, Mark Bonta explains the process his company recently accomplished as part of their goal to create a Recovery Friendly Workplace (RFW).** Mark is General Manager of Genfoot America, Inc., in Littleton. He explains the initial steps involved with taking on the Recovery Friendly Workplace Initiative. He describes the "Declaration" which serves the same purpose as the Commitment Statement for Network Organizations. He says,

...this starts with the "Declaration" to our workforce, which is one of a few initial requirements that need to be completed to receive the initial RFW designation. The next requirement is to provide training to our workforce. This training includes stigma-reduction information in most of the modules provided by the Initiative, but the most compelling is the panel of individuals that have real life experience in addiction and recovery. Employees get the opportunity to hear real stories, ask their own questions, and get to see for themselves that many of those in recovery are wonderful people. In my opinion, the most important stigma-reducing action is constant communication about recovery.

Those buried in stigma hear "Drug-Friendly-Workplace" at first, it is important to remind those people often that it is "Recovery-Friendly", not "Drug-Friendly", and Recovery is a GOOD thing. Additionally, the NH RFWI has recently partnered with OSHA (a huge step forward in the fight against negative stigma), and the Advisory Council is now seeking to forward that partnership to open communications with the insurance industry, and furthermore with Business Law.

Mark's interview continues, **please share one of your favorite quotes that describe the opportunity a Recovery-friendly workplace offers:**

That is an interesting question. **This is a new culture we are developing,** *so there are not a lot of "famous quotes" out there yet, so to pick a favorite is somewhat difficult. Instead, I'll give you two that have remained with me for some time:*

(1) *"One of the biggest challenges of kicking addiction is getting and keeping a job" and*
(2) *"Accountability is key to an individual's success in their desire to remain in recovery".*

I believe these two quotes depict the most important opportunities an RFW offers to someone in recovery: the opportunity to keep working and earning money, and to have your employer hold your job accountable to your own desire to remain in recovery.

Mark and his colleagues at Genfoot are creating a new work culture norm to support employees getting the help they need so they can keep their job and build a stable life. The prior norm was to "fire" the employee if any issue related to drug or alcohol use was addressed. This contributed to the community having to absorb those needs which increases expenses on the town. The Recovery Friendly Worksite addresses this and contributes to improving the community and strengthening families who live in the community. It is a win-win.

The Recovery Friendly Workplace began as a conversation and like any grassroots movement that meaningfully addresses a need, a single courageous conversation evolves. The North Country Task Force was established in 2018 and received expert technical assistance matching its goals with those established by the Action Collaborative for Clinician Well-Being and Resilience.

In 2019, the New Hampshire Association for Addiction Professionals (NHADACA) became the first professional association in NH to join the National Academy of Medicine Action Collaborative for Clinician Well-Being. The NHADACA Ethics Committee description and scope of purpose was updated and revised to reflect our current workforce needs and adopted the Clinician Well-Being Initiative as part of NHAHADA's strategic plan to build a resilient workforce.

The pandemic was announced in March of 2020 and has forced all of us to examine our self-care practices and adjust. These circumstances are pushing us to recognize the need to do more than lip service to the idea of wellness and being resilient.

In August of 2020, myself and other NHADACA Board members launched the first training event of the NHADACA Clinician Well-Being Initiative. Although some of the Social Distancing Protocols are being relaxed, the three-hour event was delivered on the Zoom platform. We used the Zoom Breakout Rooms for small group discussion and development of action plans to accomplish the goals of this event.

The goals for this event:

- increase awareness of the National Call to Action for Clinician Well-Being & why this is important for New Hampshire's workforce development
- invite other New Hampshire organizations and professional groups to develop a Commitment Statement, and
- become a Network Organization along with a growing number across the U.S.

One of the takeaways from this three-hour training is that talking about the problem is easy. Some of the challenges voiced during this training include, "Staff get it and want to work on these things but upper management doesn't get it," and "Our time is already consumed with putting out fires with clients". In response, we encourage participants in this training to start the conversation by sharing the resources available through the NAM Action Collaborative for clinician Well-Being and this training. These conversations will contribute to building solutions for a sustainable resilient workforce.

Invitation for Reflection and Action

How does your place of work encourage worker well-being?

Identify a few things you do for your well-being while at work:

What are your ideas for encouraging work/life balance with your co-workers? List your ideas here:

When would you put any of your ideas into action?

What else do you need to move forward with your well-being plan? List those items:

For yourself:

For your workplace:

Who will you invite to join you in this venture?

Set some target dates to help you maintain momentum

What else can you do to keep yourself engaged with this plan?

You will know your plan is working when _____

The crisis of my North Country colleague followed by my own crisis hastened my interest in examining how to be more effective at helping myself and my colleagues. Having the data from the 2018 provider needs survey verified what we already knew in our gut was not only validating but empowering.

The Summary Report was presented to the NHADACA Board of Directors at our first meeting of the new year in 2018. 96% of the respondents met at risk criteria for burnout and nearly half reported they were NOT talking about this with their boss or supervisor because they feared the loss of job security. What is more, for many of us, including myself, grinning and bearing it, putting our nose to the grindstone, and pulling up our big girl or boy pants was the work ethic norm.

The solution is simple. We need to take better care of ourselves and to do this our work culture norm needs an upgrade. Discussion began and revisions were approved to bring NHADACA's Ethics Committee description up to date and relevant to these challenges.

In 2019, NHADACA published the below Organizational Commitment Statement for Clinician Well-Being and became the first professional organization in New Hampshire to join the NAM Action Collaborative for Clinician Well-Being.

Organizational Commitment Statement

As the New Hampshire state affiliate of NAADAC, the National Association for Addiction Professionals, our mission is to provide quality education, workforce development, advocacy, ethical standards and leadership for addiction professionals. We empower efforts in prevention, treatment, and recovery. Our vision is to learn, grow, serve supporting recovery through a qualified and educated workforce.

Addiction is the number one public health issue in the United States today. Well-supported scientific evidence shows that addiction to alcohol or drugs is a chronic brain disease that has potential for recurrence and recovery. The impact of this public health issue reaches beyond Substance Use Disorder treatment professionals and across entire communities. The heart and soul of our mission is to support and nurture all practitioners: volunteers, students, interns, educators, clinicians in the community and across all health professions. We hereby commit to join with the work of the National Academy of Medicine's Action Collaborative.

We believe the health of the caregiver is an ethical imperative for assuring the integrity of our treatment systems and educational systems to insure patient care and safety. Specifically, we commit to:

- Providing current, evidence-based research and education related to chronic stress, burnout and resilience, and best practices regarding interventions at the individual, work unit, organization, and national levels.
- Bringing awareness to our members and community about the importance of self-care and taking steps to engage training opportunities to provide relevant and evidence-based tools for students, trainees, and all of our colleagues seeking to understand the disease of addiction.
- Spearheading the appropriate incorporation of integrative health practices that can reduce or prevent chronic stress and burnout and promote resilience and well-being, especially in an inter-professional setting.
- Actively participating in informing better policies on these issues.

The Seacoast Mental Health Center (SMHC) of Manchester, New Hampshire soon followed and became a Network Organization. Diane Fontneau, MS, LADC, is the Program Manager of the Substance Use Disorder treatment program services at SMHC describes her experience crafting the Commitment Statement and achieving Network Organization status for her place of employment.

From Diane Fontneau's interview: *Someone once advised me that self-care is a lifestyle not a task. I find this to be true for providing systemic change in my organization as well as in the field in general. It is not a one-time task to be accomplished, it is a daily commitment to well-being that takes on a life of its own when given the opportunity and supported by those around us.*

This is not an all or nothing commitment.

It begins with one person wanting to do one thing on one day that promotes well-being and it grows like a tree—it must be nurtured and supported, but it doesn't have to be everyone on board in order to begin taking the first step.

> Find Diane's full interview in the Turning Point
> Stories & Interview Transcripts.

None of this would have taken place without the leadership of our colleagues at the NAM Action Collaborative for Clinician Well-Being. The following statement of purpose is posted on their website page describing how to become a Network Organization. *Over the past fifty years, rates of clinician burnout have drastically increased across the United States. Clinician burnout has serious consequences for patient safety, care quality, and health care costs. The National Academy of Medicine has launched an Action Collaborative on Clinician Well-Being and Resilience to improve baseline understanding of* challenges to clinician well-being, raise visibility of clinician stress and burnout, and elevate evidence-based, multidisciplinary solutions. We invite you to join our national movement as a Network Organization.

The purpose of the Action Collaborative is to provide an opportunity for organizations across the country to discuss and share plans of action to reverse clinician burnout and promote clinician well-being. The National Academy of Medicine (NAM) has collected statements describing organizational goals or commitments to action. By sharing their commitment to improving clinician well-being and reducing clinician burnout, these organizations are an active contributor to the NAM's Action Collaborative on Clinician Well-Being and Resilience ("Network Organizations).

Instructions to organization
leaders interested in becoming a network organization
of the NAM Clinician Well-Being Collaborative:

- Draft a one- to two-page commitment statement on clinician well-being.

  o please visit NHADACA.org Clinician Well-Being page and the Network Organization webpage on the NAM Action Collaborative for Clinician Well-Being

  o you will find a list of Network Organizations and can review their Commitment Statements as examples to create your own

- You will find a "Submit a commitment statement" button. Click this button to fill out the survey and submit your own Commitment Statement on behalf of your organization

- As a network organization, your organization will be able to:

  o provide input on activities of the NAM Clinician Well-Being Collaborative.
  o receive networking and information-sharing opportunities;
  o receive regular updates on the work of the Clinician Well-Being Collaborative, including priority invitations to public meetings and advance notice of new tools and publications;
  o receive communications tools such as infographics and social media toolkits;
  o be listed on the NHADACA and NAM websites, along with the NAM Organizational "Commitment Statement" describing current and/or future work in the area of clinician well-being and a link to the NAM website; and
  o receive invitations to act as partners in building new efforts around clinician well-being at the NAM.

One of the benefits NHADACA received from becoming a Network Organization is free access to hosting their traveling art gallery: **Expressions of Clinician Well-Being.** This show was on display in the large plenary room where Dr. Arthur Hengerer, MD spoke about the Action Collaborative and some of the stories presented in the traveling art gallery during the 2019 Annual NH Behavioral Health Summit.

100 pieces of artwork were selected by a panel of reviewers to be displayed in a digital gallery. The project is part of the NAM's Action Collaborative on Clinician Well-Being and Resilience which aims to improve baseline understanding, raise the visibility of clinician stress and burnout, and elevate evidence-based, multidisciplinary solutions that will improve patient care by caring for the caregiver. To learn more, visit nam.edu/ClinicianWellBeing.

> **"The journey of a thousand miles begins with just one step"**
> *—attributed to Confucius*
>
> Quote contributed by Cynthia Thomas, PhD(c), MSN, RN
> Find Cynthia's full Turning Point Story in the Interview Transcripts.

CHAPTER NINE SUMMARY AND CONCLUSION

This final chapter concludes a full circle that began in the first chapter with the story of two trusted colleagues courageously confiding their feelings of despair about their professional practice. This initial private conversation stirred up questions including *how do we know when our practice is impaired to the point it is necessary to surrender our license?* The following year I found myself in their shoes. Thanks to my border collie Panda, her gentle intervention redirected me to put myself into psychiatric care. Fortunately, the outcomes of our stories are positive. Not only are we still alive and kicking but each of us found our way back into our zones of compassion satisfaction.

As to the answer to the original question about HOW do we maintain the precious 20% compassion satisfaction necessary to keep burnout at bay well, each of us define those details for ourselves. Each chapter walked us through the components of this answer and included lived experience testimony from interviews and Turning Point stories. Bottom line, each of us are responsible for our own well-being *and* this work ethic value needs to be integrated into our work culture norms.

Rick Hanson, author of The Neuroscience of Happiness talks about engaging our mind and body in such a way to change our brain. He calls this intentional positive neuroplasticity as outlined in the second part of the book. Put simply this means we need to be persistent with developing our ability to calm our stress response. Our breath is the one thing we are doing all the time and is the key to returning our stress response to a relaxation response through the deep diaphragmatic breathing you learned while doing **HomeBase.**

Thought leaders have studied and written their findings in the material reviewed and specific steps given by the NAM Collaborative Action for Clinician Well-Being spell out a simple process for becoming a Network Organization. The process of engaging discussion to identify and write a Commitment Statement is a mechanism for engaging courageous conversations.

What is important is for each of us to honor what we do best and care for that in a way that encourages growth in ourselves and those around us. This builds the integrity of trusted relationships and it is these relationships that carry us through our dark and our light moments.

Get involved where you thrive. If you are in a job that is not the right fit, seek out and focus on the opportunities where you can cultivate your precious 20%. Another opportunity will present itself. In doing this you will inspire others to do the same.

In closing, Tonya Tavares talks about the importance of starting the conversation. Tonya facilitated the first Technical Assistance Grant we received and was an integral part of the start-up that established the infrastructure for the North Country Task Force. As one of the managers of the Opioid Response Network, she witnessed firsthand how important it is for courageous conversations to get started. Find the full transcript of her interview in the Turning Point and Transcripts Journal.

Many citizens and professionals think they cannot make an impact regarding changing the culture of their workplace. if one of those people asked you how they could "make a difference" what would you tell them?

Tonya says, *Start the conversation. You cannot make any change or make a difference if you do not start the conversation and speak up. Then, once you have started the conversation, do something—lead by example. I tell my now 3-year-old "show me, don't just tell me"("Paulo Coelho Biography") Paulo Coelho famously said, "the world is changed by your example, not your opinion." Once you do these things, be prepared to meet resistance and tension, and have a plan for it. Anticipate what people might be feeling and why and try to understand that perspective. Once the conversation is started, encourage it and act on it; discuss and listen—really listen, and not just to their spoken words.*

Key Points from *NOT* Too Tired to Care

Chapter One: "Be kinder to yourself. And then let your kindness flood the world." Pema Chodron

20% Compassion Satisfaction keeps burnout at bay and is the part of our work we find meaning and purpose- the joy of caring.

Self-care and self-monitoring are mentioned in three of the nine Principles of the National Association for Alcohol and Drug Abuse Counselors Code of Ethics; III. Professional Responsibility and Workplace Standards, VII. Supervision and Consultation, VIII. Resolving Ethical Concerns (NAADAC).

Impaired practice is to be expected and does not necessarily mean ethical violation.

Chapter Two: "Insanity is doing the same thing over and over again and expecting different results." Albert Einstein

2018 North Country Provider Needs Assessment outcomes
96% of respondents reported at risk of burnout
Less than 45% reported receiving clinical supervision, and
are NOT talking about these symptoms because of fear they would lose their job.

Chapter Three: Necessity is the mother of invention.

According to WHO, burnout is characterized by:
Feelings of energy depletion or exhaustion
Increased mental distance from one's job, or feelings of negativism or Cynicism related to one's job, and reduced professional efficacy

Administrative leadership and workers must work together to accomplish WHO's definition of "successfully managed chronic workplace stress"

Professional quality of Life Scale (ProQOL) is a validated tool to measure Compassion Satisfaction, Burnout, and Vicarious/secondary trauma.

Chapter Four: "And acceptance is the answer to all my problems today...I need to concentrate not so much on what needs to be changed in the world as on what needs to be changed in me and my attitudes." Alcoholics Anonymous Big Book

The Green Cross Academy of Traumatology established a Code of Ethics for Self-Care. The Academy was initially organized to serve a need in Oklahoma City following the April 19, 1995 bombing of the Alfred P. Murrah Federal Building.

The Triune Brain three distinct functions: Reptilian (Instinctive drives; fight, flight, freeze), Limbic (emotions), Neocortex (rational thinking), by Paul D. MacLean, MD 1960's

The Relaxation Response: an autonomic reaction that can be stimulated using diaphragmatic breathing and activating the Vagus nerve, Herbert Benson, MD 1970;s

Chapter Five: "Emotions are like ocean waves. They rise and fall every day, every hour, and sometimes, every minute. Our job in recovery is to learn to surf the waves of our emotions, so we can stay afloat and enjoy life. If we manage our thoughts and feel our feelings, we are able to ride the waves with ease."

Quote contributed by Recovery Warriors

HomeBase is an evidence-informed practice that stimulates the vagus nerve. This nerve is important because it is a major player in the parasympathetic nervous system, which is the "rest and digest" part and functions opposite to the sympathetic nervous system which is "fight or flight".

The United States has the highest rate of incarceration in the world (937 per 100,000 adults) (Fox).

Chapter Six:

"Do what you can, where you are, with what you have." Teddy Roosevelt

*If you do not know your State Representative,
you can find their contact information by visiting
www.house.gov/representatives/find-your-
representative* then type in your zip code.

*To learn more about what you can do as a citizen to influence change,
contact* **New Futures** *603-225-9540 www.new-futures.org/our-approach*

Chapter Seven:

"Our lives begin to end the day we become silent about things that matter."

Martin Luther King, Jr.

The self-help 12-step program Alcoholics Anonymous, began in 1935.

Positive messaging campaigns such as the documentary film *The Anonymous People* and the *In Our Own Voices* program of the National Alliance for Mental Illness encourage positive culture change.

Substance Use Disorder replaced Substance Abuse and Substance Dependence in the revised edition of the Diagnostic Statistical Manual DSM5 (2013) as part of a national effort to more accurately represent this as a chronic disease, the term

Chapter Eight:

"The forces that distract the helper from vigilance can be powerful and persuasive, but we have choices. If we sort through what is happening, name it, and speak honestly about it, those choices become very clear. And decisions made in clarity can carry a sort of peace no matter what chaos surrounds us."

Pamela Woll, Compassion Doesn't Make You Tired (2019)

Any kind of change requires motivation. In terms of advocating for policy change or changes in law, being motivated is not enough. A coordinated effort is required. Laura and Elizabeth's experience illustrates the involvement and commitment required to create policy change.

Promoting self-care, Elizabeth's testimony confirms we can also experience negative effects of positive stress.

Chapter Nine:

"We cannot solve problems with the same thinking we used to create them." Albert Einstein

The Quadruple Aim model developed by the Institute of Medicine provides direction for how to improve quality of care, reduce costs, improve public health, and maintain staff well-being.

Contact your National Professional Affiliate to share resources available to Network Organizations.

Contact the National Academy of Medicine Collaborative Action on Clinician Well-Being

to learn more about what you can do and how to get involved. ClinicianWellBeing@nas.edu

The science and the researchers have given us a map and a compass for how to turn our healthcare system around. Start where you are, work with what you have, and engage your legislators with the lived experiences the data represents.

Together we can do this.

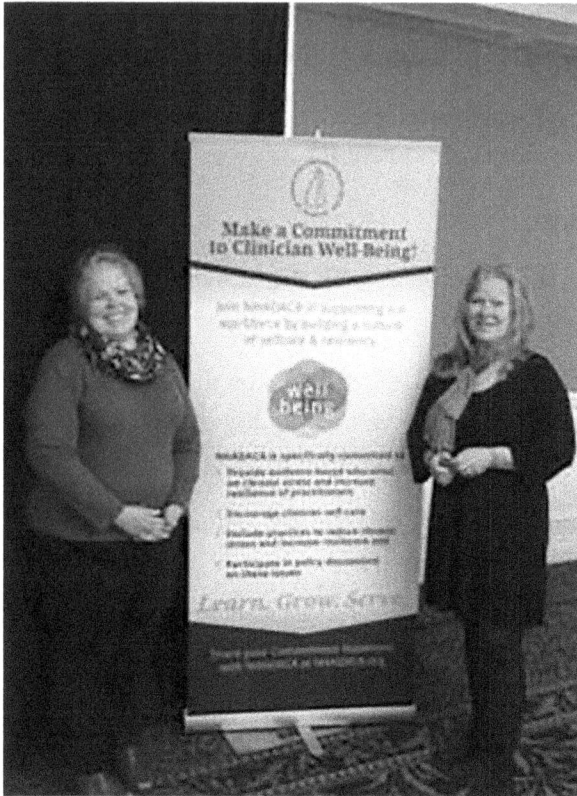

Dianne and I have our silly giggle grins on because we were so very happy to have accomplished consensus with the design of this banner.

New Hampshire Alcohol and Drug Abuse Counselors Association Clinician Well-Being Commitment Statement Banner with Executive Director, Dianne Pepin Castrucci (on the left), and Angela Thomas Jones, Chairperson Ethics Committee and North Country Region Representative

www.nhadaca.org/page-18118

EPILOGUE

Michael Meit, MA, MPH
Director of Research and Programs
ETSU Center for Rural Health Research

Megan Heffernan, MPH, Research Scientist, Public Health Research
NORC at the University of Chicago

Frances J. Feltner, DNP, MSN, RN
Director, University of Kentucky Center of Excellence in Rural Health

It is an honor to be invited to contribute to this important book. **Our charge was to offer insights and lessons learned from our work in other communities that can serve as inspiration for the stakeholders in New Hampshire that your work is making a difference.** As we think about areas that have made progress in addressing the opioid crisis, one place stands out far above others, and it may be one that surprises you. In this chapter we are going to share a story that emanates from the mountains of eastern Kentucky, deep in the heart of Appalachia—a place that shares much in common with New Hampshire in fact, from the rugged terrain to the independent spirit to the deeply ingrained pride that people have for their communities.

Why eastern Kentucky you ask? In our line of work as academic researchers we often look for **"bright spots" using** a methodology referred to as positive deviance. Essentially, we are looking for those places that, based on socio-economic and demographic factors, are doing far better than expected as compared to other similar communities. As we explored a national overdose mapping tool, the NORC Opioid Misuse Community Assessment Tool (www.opioidmisusetool.norc.org) we found a cluster of counties in eastern Kentucky where overdose rates had gone down, even as rates in similar communities in neighboring states and across the country had continued to rise. As we dug deeper, we found that among **the 10 counties in the entire United States with the steepest declines in overdose death rates** across the two time frames we explored (2008-2012 compared to 2013-2017), 8 were in eastern Kentucky. **And the rates of decline were astounding.** While the total US overdose mortality rate is around 25 deaths per 100,000 people, each of these counties saw declines that exceeded that total rate, ranging from declines of 28.8 per 100,000 to 52.2 per 100,000!

With support from the Centers for Disease Control and Prevention, and in collaboration with the National Association of County and City Health Officials, partners at the NORC Walsh Center for Rural Health Analysis and the University of Kentucky Center for Excellence in Rural Health were able to conduct a positive deviance study in eastern Kentucky to try to understand those factors that were contributing to this astounding success. Notably, despite the dramatic decreases in overdose mortality, rates in eastern Kentucky remain high, and each of those 8 counties still has a rate that exceeds that of the nation. As a result, many of the stakeholders with whom we spoke were initially surprised by our findings. As they learned more, however, that pride that is so emblematic of our Appalachian region came through. Here is some of what we learned—

- **Community coalition building makes a difference** – Early in the opioid crisis a group was organized throughout eastern Kentucky called Operation UNITE. They brought together key stakeholders, focused on community outreach and education, worked with children, positively engaged the law enforcement community, and helped individuals seek and access treatment. Their long-term, sustained effort has helped to reduce stigma within the region and has created a resource for individuals and partners wanting to make a difference in their communities. Operation UNITE has done many things for eastern Kentucky but let us say it again—their efforts have created a culture where people are empowered to seek help. They have reduced stigma within the region.

- **Access to treatment services is key** – Early on in the opioid crisis Operation UNITE served as a lifeline for individuals needing help by providing treatment vouchers that were accepted by regional treatment providers. Treatment availability took off, however, following the expansion of Medicaid within the state of Kentucky. Kentucky's Medicaid expansion included a robust substance use treatment benefit, and once services were reimbursable, treatment providers rapidly expanded treatment sites throughout the region.

- **Creation of a recovery ecosystem** – Notably, much of the treatment that is available is linked to employment training, to ensure that individuals in recovery can be successful in maintaining that recovery. Combined with robust and long-term efforts to support recovery housing and second chance employment, resources have been developed to support individuals throughout their recovery.

And of course there were other important factors as well, including efforts to limit access to the prescription drugs that formed the first wave of the opioid crisis, **a changing culture among criminal** justice officials, and the expansion of syringe services programs (SSPs) and the wide distribution of Narcan, among others. There are a few common threads across all these factors, however. First, there has **been long standing, bi-partisan support from Kentucky lawmakers**, including Governor Ernie Fletcher (R) who helped to establish the recovery housing programs, Governor Steve Beshear (D) who expanded Medicaid with that strong treatment benefit, and Representative Hal Rodgers (R) who has long been a champion for substance use prevention and treatment in the region. **Leadership matters.**

Second, change doesn't happen overnight. The work of Operation UNITE, championed by Representative Rodgers, has been 17 years in the making. Their continued focus and advocacy has created a culture shift within the region, but culture change takes time.

Finally, and most importantly, credit also goes to the people of eastern Kentucky. Not unlike those in New Hampshire, the people of Appalachia are rugged, hard-working, independent individuals. As the stigma of substance use began to fade, these strengths could be applied to working together at the community level to begin to address these issues. Rural communities also excel at community engagement, which was also evident in eastern Kentucky. Community partners from sectors including education, economic development, city and county leaders, health care, behavioral health, public health, and social services work together in a consistent manner to stay informed and find solutions.

None of this is to say that the job is done. As we noted, overdose rates remain quite high in the region, and because of COVID-19 they have been on the rise once more. In addition, as opioid use has declined, methamphetamine use has increased. To some extent that is the nature of substance use disorder. As we begin to get a handle on one drug, others emerge. That doesn't mean that this is a zero-sum game, however. What we have learned in addressing the opioid crisis can and must be applied to methamphetamine, and whatever emerges beyond that. Community engagement, advocacy, treatment availability, and development of a strong recovery ecosystem will remain key factors regardless of the substance at hand.

Here's what we want you to know. Your work is hard, and measuring change is difficult.

Those factors inevitably lead us to question our work. We know that sometimes it just feels like you are treading water. But know that your work is making a difference.

With patience and persistence, we know that progress is not only possible, it is inevitable.

BIBLIOGRAPHY AND REFERENCES

Works Cited

4th Dimension Productions. "The Anonymous People." *YouTube,* uploaded by AliveMind, 10 Dec. 2013, www.youtube.com/watch?v=bqoEtUn0Agw.

"A.A. Around the World." *Al-Anon Family Groups, 2020,* www.aa.org/pages/en_US/aa-around-the-world.

"About Brené Brown." *Brené Brown, LLC,* 2020, www.brenebrown.com/about/.

"About the CDC-Kaiser ACE Study." *Centers for Disease Control and Prevention,* 13 Apr. 2020, www.cdc.gov/violenceprevention/acestudy/about.html.

"Acupuncture Malpractice Quick Quote." *American Acupuncture Council,* 2020, www.acupuncturecouncil.com/acupuncture-malpractice-quick-quote/.

"An Ounce of Prevention is Worth a Pound of Cure." *Learning English,* 14 Mar 2020, learningenglish.voanews.com/a/an-ounce-of-prevention-is-worth-a-pound-of-cure-/5326585.html.

"APA Dictionary of Psychology." *American Psychological Association,* 2020, dictionary.apa.org/leniency-error.

"Advancing Colleague Assistance in Professional Psychology." *American Psychological Association,* 2006, www.apa.org/practice/resources/assistance/monograph.pdf.

Barnes, Haleigh, et al. "Moral Injury and PTSD: Often Co-Occurring Yet Mechanistically Different." *The Journal of Neuropsychiatry and Clinical Neurosciences,* vol. 31, no. 2, 2019, pp. A4-103.

Bernstein, Lenny. "One of the biggest challenges of kicking addiction is getting and keeping a job." *Washington Post,* 27 Nov. 2018, www.washingtonpost.com/national/health-science/one-of-the-biggest-challenges-of-kicking-addiction-is-getting-and-keeping-a-job/2018/11/27/87e8a168-d958-11e8-aeb7-ddcad4a0a54e_story.html.

Berwick, et al. "The triple aim: care, health, and cost." Health Affairs, vol. 27, no. 3, 2008, pp. 759-769.

Bodenheimer, Thomas and Christine Sinsky. "From Triple to Quadruple Aim: Care of the Patient Requires Care of the Provider." *Annals of Family Medicine,* vol. 12, no. 6, pp. 573-576, 2014, doi: 10.1370/afm.1713.

Brown, Brené, PhD, LMSW. "Brené Brown on Empathy." *Youtube,* uploaded by The RSA, 10 Dec. 2013, www.youtube.com/watch?v=1Evwgu369Jw.

"Burn-out an 'occupational phenomenon': International Classification of Diseases." *World Health Organization,* 2020, www.who.int/mental_health/evidence/burn-out/en/.

Burton, Joan. *Healthy workplaces: a model for action: for employers, workers, policymakers and practitioners.* Geneva, World Health Organization, 2010.

Cannon, Walter B. "The Wisdom of the Body." *The British Medical Journal,* vol. 2, no. 3745, 1932.

Carrico, Mara. "A Beginner's Guide to the History of Yoga." *Yoga Journal,* 22 May 2017, www.yogajournal.com/yoga-101/the-roots-of-yoga.

Carroll, Roger. "A Journey Through NH's Mental Health System." *Granite State News Collaborative,* 24 Apr. 2019, www.collaborativenh.org/solutionstories/2019/1/5/a-journey-through-nhs-mental-health-system-hldng.

Carroll, Roger. "A Journey Through NH's Mental Health System, Part 1 of 3." *The Laconia Daily Sun,* 24 Dec. 2018, www.laconiadailysun.com/news/local/a-journey-through-nhs-mental-health-system-part-1-of-3/article_cc9a152e-07cc-11e9-b23c-1f08564fdf18.html.

Centers for Disease Control and Prevention. National Center for Injury Prevention and Control, Division of Violence Prevention, 2020, www.cdc.gov/violenceprevention/acestudy/about.html.

Chao, Maria T., et al. "Utilization of Group-Based, Community Acupuncture Clinics: A Comparative Study with a Nationally Representative Sample of Acupuncture Users." *Journal of Alternative and Complementary Medicine,* vol. 18, no. 6, Jun. 2012, ncbi.nlm.nih.gov/pmc/articles/PMC3390970/.

Chatterjee, Rhitu and Carmel Wroth. "WHO Redefines Burnout As A 'Syndrome' Linked To Chronic Stress At Work." *WBUR News,* 28 May 2019, www.wbur.org/npr/727637944/who-redefines-burnout-as-a-syndrome-linked-to-chronic-stress-at-work.

Clare, Bevin A., et al. "The Diuretic Effect in Human Subjects of an Extract of *Taraxacum officinale* Folium over a Single Day." *The Journal of Alternative and Complementary Medicine,* vol. 15, no. 8, 2009, doi.org/10.1089/acm.2008.0152.

Clay, Rebecca A. "COVID-19 and suicide." *American Psychological Association,* 1 Jun. 2020, www.apa.org/monitor/2020/06/covid-suicide.

"Continuum of Care." *New Hampshire Department of Health and Human Services,* 2016, www.dhhs.nh.gov/dcbcs/bdas/continuum-of-care.htm.

Cooley, Laura, LAc. "Unimagined Bridges." *Youtube,* uploaded by acuaid, 19 May 2011, www.youtube.com/watch?v=7C7NzqB7p3s&fbclid= IwAR3G5fEH_iuoqjxsBlLKZIvFe4uT80fhpmohN4cte4vpSOB_ 6M5_drHCQgs.

Cronin, Mike. "Parents of suspected overdose victims hope their son's story helps others." *WMUR9,* 15 Mar. 2016, www.wmur.com/article/parents-of-suspected-overdose-victim-hope-son-s-story-helps-others/5209411#.

Cudmore, Becca. "The Evolutionary Roots of Instinct." *The Scientist,* 16 Jul. 2017, www.the-scientist.com/notebook/the-evolutionary-roots-of-instinct-31217.

Davidson, Helen. "Chinese inquiry exonerates coronavirus whistleblower doctor." *The Guardian,* 20 Mar. 2020, www.theguardian.com/world/2020/mar/20/chinese-inquiry-Exonerates-coronavirus-whistleblower-doctor-li-wenliang.

"Depression: What is burnout?" *Institute for Quality and Efficiency in Health Care,* 2020, www.ncbi.nlm.nih.gov/books/NBK279286/.

Diagnostic and Statistical Manual of Mental Disorders. 5th ed., American Psychiatric Association, 2013.

DiClemente, Carlo C., and James O. Prochaska. "Toward a comprehensive, transtheoretical model of change: Stages of change and addictive behaviors." *Applied clinical psychology. Treating addictive behaviors,* 1998, doi.org/10.1007/978-1-4899-1934-2_1.

Drapeau, C. W., and J. L. McIntosh. "U.S.A. Suicide: 2018 Official Final Data." *American Association of Suicidology,* 2020, suicidology.org/wp-content/uploads/2020/02/2018datapgsv2_Final.pdf.

"Dr. Rick Hanson: The Neuroscience of Lasting Happiness." *Rick Hanson, PhD,* 2020, www.rickhanson.net/.

Dzau, Victor J., M.D., et al. "Preventing a Parallel Pandemic — A National Strategy to Protect Clinicians' Well-Being." *The New England Journal of Medicine,* vol. 383, 2020, pp. 513-515, www.nejm.org/doi/full/10.1056/NEJMp2011027.

Dzau, Victor J., M.D., et al. "To Care is Human: Collectively Confronting the Clinician-Burnout Crisis." *The New England Journal of Medicine,* vol. 378, no. 4, 2018, pp. 312-314, med.emory.edu/departments/medicine/_documents/caring-is-human.pdf.

Encouraging the Well-Being and Recovery of NH Health Care Professionals through Compassion, Education, Advocacy, Hope. New Hampshire Professionals Health Program. 2020, www.nhphp.org/.

"Expressions of Clinician Well-Being." *National Academy of Medicine.* 2020, nam.edu/expressions-of-clinician-well-being-an-art-exhibition/.

"Facing Addiction in America: The Surgeon General's Report on Alcohol, Drugs, and Health." *U.S. Department of Health and Human Services, Office of the Surgeon General,* 2016, addiction.surgeongeneral.gov/sites/default/files/surgeon-generals-report.pdf.

"Fatigue in the Workplace." *American Psychological Association.* Vol. 69, No.2, June 2017. www.apa.org/pubs/journals/special/5516902

"FAQ About Al-Anon's history." *Al-Anon Family Groups,* 2020, al-anon.org/for-members/wso/archives/faq-al-anons-history.

Feeley, Derek. "The Triple Aim or the Quadruple Aim? Four Points to Help Set Your Strategy." *Institute for Healthcare Improvement,* 28 Nov. 2017, www.ihi.org/communities/blogs/the-triple-aim-or-the-quadruple-aim-four-points-to-help-set-your-strategy.

Feldman, Nina, WHYY. "Pandemic Presents New Hurdles, And Hope, For People Struggling With Addiction." *Kaiser Health News,* 2 Jun. 2020, khn.org/news/pandemic-presents-new-hurdles-and-hope-for-people-struggling-with-addiction/.

Felitti, Vincent J., MD, FACP, et al. "Relationship of Childhood Abuse and Household Dysfunction to Many of the Leading Causes of Death in Adults: The Adverse Childhood Experiences (ACE) Study." *American Journal of Preventive Medicine,* vol. 14, no. 4, 1998, www.ajpmonline.org/article/S0749-3797(98)00017-8/abstract.

"Fentanyl and Carfentanil." *Ottawa Public Health,* 3 Mar. 2020, www.ottawapublichealth.ca/en/public-health-topics/fentanyl-and-carfentanil.aspx.

Figley, Charles L. *Stress Disorders Among Vietnam Veterans: Theory, Research,* Brunner-Routledge, 1978.

"Founder Clara Barton." *American Red Cross,* 2020, www.redcross.org/content/dam/redcross/enterprise-assets/about-us/history/history-clara-barton-v3.pdf.

Fox, Aaron D., et al. "Release from incarceration, relapse to opioid use and the potential for buprenorphine maintenance treatment: a qualitative study of the perceptions of former inmates with opioid use disorder." *Addiction Science and Clinical Practice,* vol. 10, no. 2, 2015, doi.org/10.1186/s13722-014-0023-0.

Friedberg, Mark W. "Factors Affecting Physician Professional Satisfaction and Their Implications for Patient Care, Health Systems, and Health Policy." *RAND Corporation,* 2013, www.rand.org/pubs/research_reports/RR439. html.

"GNYHA Tackles Clinician Burnout in Hospitals." *Greater New York Hospital Association,* 16 Apr. 2018, www.gnyha.org/news/gnyha-tackles-clinician-burnout-in-hospitals.

Granite State News Collaborative. 2020, www.collaborativenh.org/.

"Green Cross." *Charles R. Figley,* charlesfigley.com/green-cross.

Healthy workplaces: a model for action. World Health Organization, 2010.

Hengerer, Arthur, and Sandeep P. Kishore. "Breaking a Culture of Silence: The Role of State Medical Boards." *National Academy of Medicine,* 28 Aug. 2017, nam. edu/breaking-a-culture-of-silence-the-role-of-state-medical-boards/.

"Historical Data: The Birth of A.A. and Its Growth in the U.S./Canada." *Al-Anon Family Groups, 2020,* www.aa.org/pages/en_US/historical-data-the-birth-of-aa-and-its-growth-in-the-uscanada.

"How long did Prohibition last?" *Encyclopaedia Britannica,* 2020, www.britannica.com/story/how-long-did-prohibition-last.

Itchhaporia, Dipti. "The Quadruple Aim." *American College of Cardiology,* April 26, 2018, www.acc.org/membership/sections-and-councils/cardiovascular-management-section/section-updates/2018/04/26/12/07/the-quadruple-aim.

"International Statistical Classification of Diseases and Related Health Problems 10th Revision." *World Health Organization,* 2016, icd.who.int/browse10/2016/en.

Jameton, Andrew. *Nursing practice: the ethical issues.* Prentice-Hall, 1984.

"John L. Lewis." *AFL-CIO, America's Unions,* 2020, aflcio.org/about/history/labor-history-people/john-lewis.

Lad, Vasant, BAM & S, MASc. "Ayurveda: A Brief Introduction And Guide." *The Ayurvedic Institute,* 2020 www.ayurveda.com/resources/articles/ayurveda-a-brief-introduction-and-guide.

Lanese, Nicoletta. "What is Homeostasis?" *Live Science,* 15 July 2019, www.livescience.com/65938-homeostasis.html.

Lewis, Sandra J., et al. "Changes in the Professional Lives of Cardiologists Over 2 Decades." *Journal of the American College of Cardiology,* vol. 69, no. 4, pp. 452-462, Jan. 2017, DOI: 10.1016/j.jacc.2016.11.027.

Manzo, Lynne C., and Patrick Devine-Wright. *Place Attachment: Advances in Theory, Methods and Applications.* Routledge, 2013.

Masero, Monica. "The Wisdom of the Body and Couple Therapy – A Sensorimotor Psychotherapy Perspective: An Interview with Pat Ogden." *Australian and New Zealand Journal of Family Therapy*, 15 Dec. 2017, doi.org/10.1002/anzf.1267.

Maslow, Abraham H. "Toward a Psychology of Being." 1962, en.wiktionary.org/wiki/if_all_you_have_is_a_hammer,_everything_looks_like_a_nail.

Mealer, Meredith M., et al. "Increased prevalence of post-traumatic stress disorder symptoms in critical care nurses." *American Journal of Respiratory and Critical Care Medicine*, vol. 175, no. 7, 2007, pp. 693-697.

"Medication-Assisted Treatment (MAT)." *Substance Abuse and Mental Health Services Administration,* 1 Sept. 2019, www.samhsa.gov/medication-assisted-treatment.

"Mirror Neurons and the Benefits of Community Acupuncture." People's Organization of Community Acupuncture, 2020, www.pocacoop.com/prick-prod-provoke/post/mirror-neurons-and-the-benefits-of-community-acupuncture.

Mount Washington Observatory. 2020, www.mountwashington.org.

Mount Washington. Wikipedia, 2020, en.wikipedia.org/wiki/Mount_Washington.

NAADAC, The Association for Addiction Professionals. NAADAC/NCC AP Code of Ethics, 2020, www.naadac.org/assets/2416/naadac-code-of-ethics-033117.pdf.

"NAMI In Our Own Voice." *National Alliance on Mental Illness,* 2020, www.nami.org/Support-Education/Mental-Health-Education/NAMI-In-Our-Own-Voice.

NARCAN. Emergent BioSolutions Inc., 2020, www.narcan.com/community/education-awareness-and-training-resources/#isi_anchor.

National Academy of Medicine. National Academy of Sciences, 2020, nam.edu/initiatives/clinician-resilience-and-well-being.

National Acupuncture Detoxification Association. NADA, 2020, acudetox.com/about-nada/

"National Mental Health Survey of Doctors and Medical Students." *Beyondblue: Depression. Anxiety.* 2013, www.beyondblue.org.au/docs/default-source/research-project-files/bl1132-report—nmhdmss-full-report_web.

"New Hampshire Behavioral Health Summit." *New Hampshire Behavioral Health Summit 2020,* 2020, www.nhbhs.com/.

"New Hampshire Juvenile Resources Manual." *The Judicial Planning Committee, New Hampshire Supreme Court,* 1978, www.ncjrs.gov/pdf-files1/Digitization/65219NCJRS.pdf.

"Network Organizations of the Action Collaborative on Clinician Well-Being and Resilience." *National Academy of Medicine,* 2020, nam.edu/action-collaborative-on-clinician-well-being-and-resilience-network-organizations/.

Nguyen, Steve, PhD. "In Chinese: Crisis Does Not Mean Danger and Opportunity." *Workplace Psychology,* 10 Aug. 2014, workplacepsychology.net/2014/08/10/in-chinese-crisis-does-not-mean-danger-and-opportunity/.

NH Division of Forests and Lands. State of New Hampshire, 2019, www.nh.gov/nhdfl/reports/forest-statistics.htm.

"NH family uses son's overdose death as moment to tackle opioid crisis." *WCVB5,* 11 Mar. 2016, www.wcvb.com/article/nh-family-uses-son-s-overdose-death-as-moment-to-tackle-opioid-crisis/8232616#.

NIDA. "Heroin DrugFacts." *National Institute on Drug Abuse,* 21 Nov. 2019, www.drugabuse.gov/publications/drugfacs/heroin.

O'Connor, Michael F., PhD. "Intervening with an Impaired Colleague." *American Psychological Association Services, Inc.,* 2008, www.apaservices.org/practice/ce/self-care/intervening#:~:text=Ethical%20Responsibilities,is%20thought%20to%20be%20impaired.&text=Impairment%20therefore%20refers%20to%20circumstances,professional%20services%20by%20the%20psychologist.

Onyett, Steve, et al. "Job satisfaction and burnout among members of community mental health teams." *Journal of Mental Health,* vol. 6, no. 1, 1997, psycnet.apa.org/record/1997-08103-007.

Opioid Response Network. 2018, www.opioidresponsenetwork.org/.

"Ounce of Prevention, Pound of Cure." *University of Cambridge,* 9 Oct. 2012, www.cam.ac.uk/research/news/ounce-of-prevention-pound-of-cure.

"Overview of Vivitrol (Naltrexone)." *American Addiction Centers,* 4 Feb. 2020, www.americanaddictioncenters.org/addiction-medications/vivitrol.

"Panic Attack on Live Television." *Youtube,* uploaded by ABC News, 10 Mar. 2014, https://www.youtube.com/watch?v=_qo4uPxhUzU&index=9&t=0s&list=PLdfDJIUx4wgmupDbvWKFW0uHo3WKX80SE.

"Paulo Coelho Biography." *Biography.* 9 Nov. 2019, www.biography.com/writer/paulo-coelho.

Porges, Stephen W. *The Polyvagal Theory: Neurophysiological Foundations of Emotions, Attachment, Communication, Self-Regulation.* W. W. Norton and Company, 2011.

"PQC Works." *PQC,* 2020, pqcworks.com/pqc-works/.

"Professional Quality of Life Measure." *The Center for Victims of Torure,* 2019, proqol.org/Compassion_Satisfaction.html.

"Protecting Veterans' Access to Mental Health Care." *National Alliance on Mental Illness,* 2020, www.nami.org/Advocacy/Policy-Priorities/Improve-Care/Protecting-Veterans-Access-to-Mental-Health-Care.

"QD85 Burn-out." *ICD-11 for Mortality and Morbidity Statistics,* 2019, icd.who.int/browse11/l-m/en#/http://id.who.int/icd/entity/129180281.

"QuickFacts, New Hampshire." *United States Census Bureau,* 2019, www.census.gov/quickfacts/NH.

"Quick Covid-19 Primary Care Survey." *Primary Care Collaborative,* 13 Jul. 2020, static1.squarespace.com/static/5d7ff8184cf0e01e4566cb02/t/5f1a-f2ac7d6bfd1787ad68f2/1595601581976/C19+Series+16+National+Executive+Summary.pdf.

"Recovery and Recovery Support." *Substance Abuse and Mental Health Services Administration,* 23 Apr. 2020, www.samhsa.gov/find-help/recovery.

Ren. "Prison Sentences Don't Help Drug Addicts — A Look at Post-Prison Relapse Rates." *Narconon,* 28 Feb. 2020, www.narconon.org/blog/prison-sentences-dont-help-drug-addicts-a-look-at-post-prison-relapse-rates.html.

Shanafelt, Tait D., MD, et al. "Career fit and burnout among academic faculty." Archives of internal medicine, vol. 169,10 (2009): 990-5. doi:10.1001/archinternmed.2009.70.

Shanafelt, Tait D., MD, and John H. Noseworthy, MD, CEO. "Executive Leadership and Physical Well-being." *Mayo Clinic Proceedings,* vol. 92, no. 1, 2016, pp. 129-146.

Shay, Jonathan, and James Munroe. "Group and milieu therapy for veterans with complex posttraumatic stress disorder." *Posttraumatic stress disorder: A comprehensive text,* Allyn and Bacon, 1998, pp. 391-413.

Sipherd, Ray. "The third-leading cause of death in US most doctors don't want you to know about." *CNBC: Modern Medicine,* 22 Feb. 2018, www.

cnbc.com/2018/02/22/medical-errors-third-leading-cause-of-death-in-america.html.

Skerrett, Patrick J. "Suicide often not preceded by warnings." *Harvard Health Publishing,* 2019, www.health.harvard.edu/blog/suicide-often-not-preceded-by-warnings-201209245331.

Stallings, Erika. "California's 1st Surgeon General Spotlights Health Risks Of Childhood Adversity." *NPR: Houston Public Media,* 2019, www.npr.org/sections/health-shots/2019/07/02/733896346.

Stamm, Beth Hudnall. "Professional Quality of Life: Compassion Satisfaction and Fatigue Version 5 (ProQOL)", 2012, www.proqol.org.

Stedman, Richard C. "Toward a Social Psychology of Place: Predicting Behavior from Place-Based Cognitions, Attitude, and Identity." *Sage Journals,* vol. 34, no. 5, pp. 561-581, 1 Sept. 2002, doi.org/10.1177/0013916502034005001.

Substance Abuse and Mental Health Services Administration. "Screening and Assessment of Co-occurring Disorders in the Justice System." Substance Abuse and Mental Health Services Administration, 2015, store.samhsa.gov/sites/default/files/d7/priv/pep19-screen-codjs.pdf.

"Suicide and Occupation." *Centers for Disease Control and Prevention,* 2019, www.cdc.gov/niosh/topics/stress/suicide.html.

"Standards of Care." *Green Cross Academy of Traumatology,* greencross.org/about-gc/standards-of-care-guidelines/.

Talbot, Simon G., and Wendy Dean. "Physicians aren't 'burning out.' They're suffering from moral injury."

STAT, 26 July 2018, www.statnews.com/2018/07/26/physicians-not-burning-out-they-are-suffering-moral-injury/.

Teater, Martha, and John Ludgate. *Overcoming Compassion Fatigue: A Practical Resilience Workbook.* PESI Publishing and Media, 2014.

Ten Percent Happier Podcast with Dan Harris. Ten Percent Happier, 2020, www.tenpercent.com/work.

The Anonymous People. Directed by Greg Williams, 4th Dimension Products, 2013.

"The Big Book (Alcoholics Anonymous)." *Wikipedia,* 30 Jul. 2020, en.wikipedia.org/wiki/The_Big_Book_(Alcoholics_Anonymous).

"The Employee Burnout Crisis: Study Reveals Big Workplace Challenge in 2017." *Kronos Incorporated,* 9 Jan 2017, www.kronos.com/about-us/newsroom/employeeburnout-crisis-study-reveals-big-workplace-challenge-2017.

"The New Hampshire House of Representatives." *The New Hampshire General Court,* 2018, www.gencourt.state.nh.us/house/members/member.aspx?member=377064.

"The Stress-Distress-Impairment Continuum for Psychologists." *American Psychological Association Services, Inc.,* 2020, www.apaservices.org/practice/ce/self-care/colleague-assist.

"To Err is Human: Building a Safer Health System." *National Academy of Sciences,* Nov. 1999, www.nap.edu/resource/9728/To-Err-is-Human-1999--report-brief.pdf.

"Tradition Two: Group Conscience or Mob Rule?" *Big Book Sponsorship,* 2020, www.bigbooksponsorship.org/articles-alcoholism-addic-tion-12-step-program-recovery/twelve-traditions-group-conscience-mob-rule/tradition-group-conscience-mob-rule/.

Turner, Ashley. "Stress and rigorous work schedules push a doctor to commit suicide every day in the US: 'We need them, but they need us'." *CNBC Healthy Returns,* 21 May 2019, www.cnbc.com/2019/ 05/21/stress-and-rigorous-work-push-a-doctor-to-commit-suicide-every-day-in-us.html.

To Err is Human. Directed by Mike Eisenberg, Tall Tale Productions, 2018.

"Trust Your Gut." *PQC,* 9 Sep. 2019, pqcworks.com/trust-your-gut/.

"Understanding Anonymity." *Alcoholics Anonymous,* 2011, www.aa.org/pages/en_US/understanding-anonymity.

Valentine, C. Michael. "Tackling the Quadruple Aim." *Journal of the American College of Cardiology,* vol. 71, no. 15, Apr. 2018, DOI: 10.1016/j.jacc.2018.03.014.

Weiner, Stacy. "COVID-19 and the opioid crisis: When a pandemic and an epidemic collide." *AAMC,* 27 Jul. 2020, www.aamc.org/news-insights/covid-19-and-opioid-crisis-when-pandemic- And-epidemic-collide.

"What is Green Cross? The Difference Between the Green Cross and the Red Cross!" *Profarma,* 2014, www.profarma.al/index.php/news-and-media-profarma/blog/174-what-is-green-cross-the-differEnce-between-the-green-cross-and-the-red-cross.

White, William. "The History and Future of Peer-based Addiction Recovery Support Services." 2004, www.williamwhitepapers.com/pr/2004Peer RecoverySupportServices.pdf.

"WHO Redefines Burnout As A 'Syndrome' Linked To Chronic Stress At Work." *NPR, Houston Public Media, 2019,* www.npr.org/sections/

health-shots/2019/05/28/727637944/who-redefines-burnout-as-a-syndrome-linked-to-chronic-stress-at-work. Accessed 29 May 2019.

Wolchover, Natalie. "The 7 Biggest Mysteries of the Human Body." *Live Science,* 27 July 2012, www.livescience.com/34095-biggest-mysteries-human-body.html.

Woll, Pamela. "Compassion Doesn't Make You Tired!" *Addiction Technology Transfer Center Network,* 2019, attcnetwork.org/sites/default/files/2019-05/Compassion-Doesnt-Make-You-Tired- NCO.pdf.

"Working Together to Connect New Hampshire." *Granite State News Collaborative,* 2020, www.collaborativenh.org/.

"Young and Sober in A.A.: From Drinking to Recovery." *Al-Anon Family Groups, 2020,* www.aa.org/pages/en_US/index.

Zimmer, Benjamin. "Crisis = Danger + Opportunity: The Plot Thickens." *Language Log,* 27 Mar. 2007, itre.cis.upenn.edu/~myl/languagelog/archives/004343.html.

You are braver than you believe,

Stronger than you seem,

And smarter than you think.

- Winnie the Pooh

BIOGRAPHIES & CONTACT INFORMATION FROM THE INTERVIEWS

Keith Anderson, LADC, Owner and Operator White Mountain Recovery Homes in Littleton, New Hampshire. 669 Union Street Littleton, NH www.whitemountainsrecovery.com/

Mark Bonta, Genfoot Plant Manager, Littleton, NH www.linkedin.com/in/mark-bonta
Recovery Friendly Advisor NH Governor's Recovery Friendly Workplace.

Elaine Davis, MS, LCMHC, MLADC co-lead of the Health Care Workgroup of the North Country Task Force investigating more effective Supervision practices for addiction treatment workforce development. She is currently a New Hampshire Department of Health and Human Services Consultant and operates a small private practice. daviselaine0@gmail.com

Doris Enman, MS, CRSW Executive Director North Country Serenity Recovery Support Center in Littleton, New Hampshire. 45 Union St, Littleton, NH 03561. (phone) 603-444-1300
www.nhrecoveryhub.org/find-help/north-country-serenity-center

Diane Fontneau, MS, LADC Seacoast SUD Program Manager
New Hampshire Alcohol and Drug Abuse Counselors Association (NHADACA) Student Representative.

Dr. Sally Garhart, MD Medical Director New Hampshire Professional Health Program (NHPHP) www.nhphp.org/ 125 Airport Rd, Concord, NH 03301. Mailing Address: PO Box 6274, Amherst, NH 0303. (603) 491-5036 sgarhart@nhphp.org

Diana Gibbs, MHA North Country Health Consortium
At Large Board Member of NH Alcohol and Drug Abuse Counselors Association (NHADACA) dgibbs@nchcnh.org

Shelly Golden, MSW, Coordinator Grafton County Mental Health Court in New Hampshire. She is the liaison to connect mentally ill offenders with mental health courts through the Grafton County Department of Corrections. www.co.grafton.nh.us/all-departments/alternative-sentencing/mental-health-court/

Samantha Lewandowski, MS Recovery Friendly Advisor New Hampshire Governor's Recovery Friendly Workplace, Concord, New Hampshire. www.recoveryfriendlyworkplace.com/team

Rebecca Libby, MA has worked as a School Counselor for the Manchester School District for nearly two decades and teaches online courses in counseling psychology for Southern New Hampshire University. rlibby@mansd.org

Linda Massimilla, Vice-Chair States/Federal Relations and Veterans Affairs Committee Grafton 1 New Hampshire State Representative. balloontraveler@yahoo.com

Karen McNamara, LADC, SAP Board of Directors member for the North Country Serenity Center Recovery Support Center. She has provided contracted clinical services for the New Hampshire State Prison and the Grafton County Department of Corrections for two decades. www.karenmcnamaraladc.com/

Elizabeth Ropp, Licensed Community Acupuncturist, Manchester Acupuncture Studio in Manchester, New Hampshire. www.manchesteracupuncturestudio.org/

Lara Saffo, Esq former Grafton County Prosecuting Attorney

Tonya Tavares, MS, CCRP, Assistant Project Director, Center for Alcohol and Addictions Studies, Brown University School of Public Health; Technology Transfer Specialist, Opioid Response Network STR-TA, New England Region 1- CT, MA, ME, NH, RI, VT. www.linkedin.com/in/tonya-tavares-2b28bb9/

Sue Thistle, MS, MLADC, North Country Task Force Policy and Administration Workgroup

New Hampshire Alcohol and Drug Abuse Counselors Association (NHADACA) Policy Committee Chairperson. Best Selling Author, Chem-Free Sobriety: 101 Trailblazers share wisdom (2020).

Cynthia Thomas, PhD(c), MSN, RN is Program Chair, Nursing Education at Western Governors University with more than 40-years of experience in program development, leadership, population health management, and higher education. cthomas1414@gmail.com

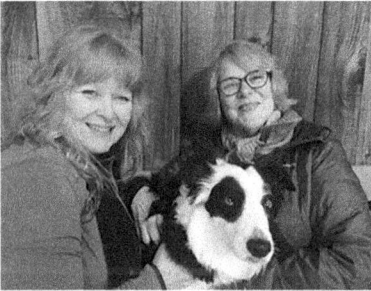

Panda
with
sistah power
Angela and Cynthia
at home in
Bethlehem, New Hampshire

ABOUT THE AUTHOR

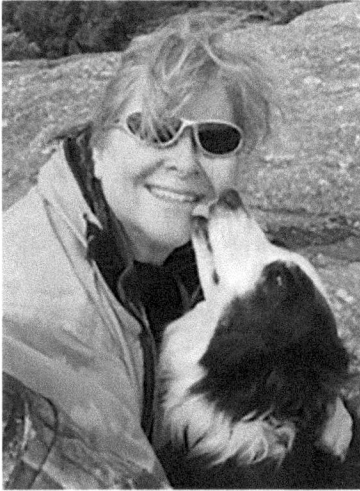

Angela and Registered Therapy Dog Panda
on Artist's Bluff, 2,014.00 ft
Franconia Notch, New Hampshire.

Angela Thomas Jones travels coast to coast presenting and teaching others resilient work-life balance for the individual and the organization. She is certified as a Compassion Fatigue Professional, specializes in trauma-sensitive mind-body practices, and registered as a Therapy Dog Handler. She is licensed in New Hampshire as a Mental Health Counselor and master's level Addiction Professional as well as a Clinical Supervisor with three decades of experience. In her service on the Board of Directors of the New Hampshire Alcohol and Drug Abuse Counselors Association (NHADACA) as the North Country Region Representative and Chairperson of the Ethics Committee she spearheaded re-defining the role of the Ethics Committee based on data showing a large number of clinicians and healthcare workers are burned out and not talking about this in the workplace because of fear they would lose their job. In 2019, NHADACA became the first addiction treatment professional association in the United States to become a Network Organization with the National Academy of Medicine's Action Collaborative for Clinician Well-being and Resilience. In 2020, she worked with her NHADACA colleagues to launch a series of remote training to enable other organizations to join this national movement and transform the burnout work culture norms into a thriving and resilient workforce culture. Angela consults with other programs and organizations to cultivate their niche in this national movement. Originally born and raised in southwestern Virginia, she and her husband live in the North Country of New Hampshire where they raised their family and continue to enjoy New England's long snowy winters. Angela also enjoys backyard herbalism, beekeeping, being in the woods during all four seasons, and living a simple life in the mountains.

URGENT PLEA!

Thank You for Reading My Book!

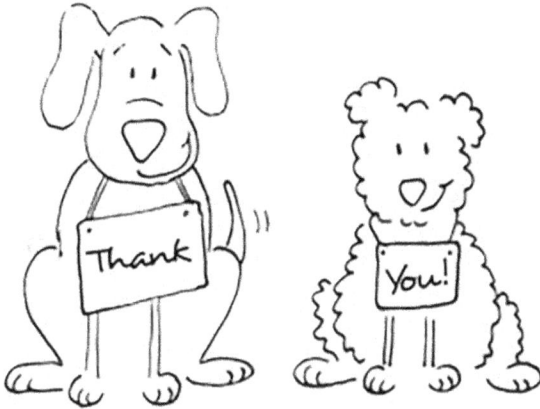

I really appreciate all of your feedback, and
I love hearing what you have to say.
I need your input to make the next version of this book and
my future books better.
Please leave me a helpful review on Amazon letting me
know what you thought of the book.
Thanks so much!!

- Angela and Panda